W9-DEK-791

ARTERIES IN CLINICAL HYPERTENSION

ARTERIES IN CLINICAL HYPERTENSION

Michel E. Safar

Department of Internal Medicine and INSERM (U 337)
Broussais Hospital
Paris, France

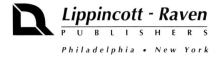

Lippincott - Raven
PUBLISHERS
Philadelphia • New York

6   5   4   3   2   1

Library of Congress Cataloging-in-Publication Data

Safar, Michel.
   Arteries in clinical hypertension / by Michel Safar.
      p.   cm.
   Includes bibliographical references and index.
   ISBN 0-397-51484-0
   1. Hypertension—Pathophysiology.   2. Arteries—Pathophysiology.
   I. Title.
   [DNLM: 1. Hypertension—physiopathology.   2. Arteries—
   physiopathology.   3. Arteries—drug effects.   4. Antihypertensive
   Agents.   WG 340 S128a 1996]
   RC685.H8S234   1994
   616. 1'32—dc20
   DNLM/DLC
   for Library of Congress   94-16167

The material contained in this volume was submitted as previously unpublished material, except in the instances in which credit has been given to the source from which some of the illustrative material was derived.

Great care has been taken to maintain the accuracy of the information contained in the volume. However, neither Lippincott–Raven Publishers nor the editors can be held responsible for errors or for any consequences arising from the use of the information herein.

The authors and publisher have exerted every effort to ensure that drug selection and dosage set forth in this text are in accord with current recommendations and practice at the time of publication. However, in view of ongoing research, changes in government regulations, and the constant flow of information relating to drug therapy and drug reactions, the reader is urged to check the package insert for each drug for any change in indications and dosage and for added warnings and precautions. This is particularly important when the recommended agent is a new or infrequently employed drug.

Materials appearing in this book prepared by individuals as part of their official duties as U.S. Government employees are not covered by the above mentioned copyright.

PREFACE

In past years, the basic knowledge of hypertension in humans has expanded not only from a better understanding of its pathophysiology but also from the clinical use of new antihypertensive agents, which were introduced somewhat independently from the studies of the mechanisms of hypertension. The advances in antihypertensive drugs were an important teaching for clinical investigators. It became apparent that even with effective treatment, complications could occur in cases of hypertension, mostly affecting the large arteries, particularly the coronary arteries.

In this respect, the concept has been developed by which the level of blood pressure in hypertension is influenced not only by increased total peripheral resistance and constriction of small arteries but also by the stiffness of large arteries. The latter condition, which involves a disproportionate increase in systolic pressure over diastolic pressure, poses a particularly serious problem because elevations of mean pressure and peripheral resistance are associated with evidence of large artery hardening. Out of this basic assumption has grown an extensive investigation of the large arteries, an approach previously not taken into major consideration in the field of hypertension. Because hypertensive vascular disease has been clinically described in a more general epidemiological framework, documenting its effects on cardiovascular morbidity and mortality, large artery disturbances can now be included within the definition of hypertension, independent of the aging and atherosclerotic processes.

From this book the reader might gain the impression that several aspects of hypertension have been largely neglected. However, in judging, the reader must consider two points. First, experimental aspects not corroborated by associated clinical evidence have been excluded from the review. Second, in several cases it may be difficult to differentiate between secondary and primary hypertension in humans, and the exclusive purpose of the book was to describe the arterial aspects of essential hypertension in adults. Finally, the fields of research are so extensive that it is almost impossible to present a complete overview of the problems. Our purpose was rather to stimulate the reader with a reasonable discussion, even if the pedagogic aspects were dismissed in some instances; this goal was particularly emphasized in the conclusion of the book which is based on a critical review of the therapeutic trials of hypertension.

Michel E. Safar

Acknowledgments

Not a single chapter could have been written without several friends who worked with me for many years, such as Drs. London, Laurent, Benetos, Asmar, and Pannier. I would also like to recognize my debt to the institutions that have helped me through the years: *l'Assistance Publique de Paris* and *l'Institut National de la Santé et de la Recherche Médicale* (INSERM). Mrs. Seban took charge of the secretarial detail, and I am particularly grateful for her extensive contribution.

The publication of this book was made possible through a grant from Groupe de Recherche Servier.

Contents

Chapter 1

Introduction: The Arterial System and the Definition of   1
Hypertension

    The arbitrary definition of hypertension   1
    Fourier analysis of the blood pressure curve   2
    The definition of hypertension on the basis of increased mean
        arterial pressure   5
    The arteries as an important bias in the research of
        hypertension   7

SECTION I

Arteries in Untreated Clinical Hypertension

Chapter 2

The Arterial System: Simplified Basic Concepts   11

    The function of arteries   11
    The pressure-volume relationship   13
    Geometry versus mechanics   16
    Appendix: The stress-strain relationship   17

Chapter 3

Pulsatile Pressure and Hypertension in Large Arteries   21

    The pulsatile component   21
    Wave reflections and hypertension   25

CHAPTER 4

Cross-Sectional Area, Stiffness, and Thickness of the   *31*
Large Arteries in Hypertension

   Cross-sectional area and diameter changes   31
   Indices of arterial stiffness in subjects with hypertension   35
   Arterial thickening and structural changes   40
   An overview   44

SECTION II
Large Arteries and Antihypertensive Drug Treatment

CHAPTER 5

Pharmacological Effects of Antihypertensive Agents   *49*
on the Arteries

   Simplified basic concepts   49
   Converting enzyme inhibitors   50
   Calcium-entry blockers   52
   Nitrates and derivatives   53
   Alpha- and beta-adrenergic blocking agents   54
   Sodium- and diuretic-induced changes in arterial diameter
      and stiffness   56
   Drug-induced change in wave reflections   58
   A simple overview of the arterial changes produced by
      antihypertensive agents   60

CHAPTER 6

Arteries and Long-Term Antihypertensive Therapy   *61*

   Structural changes of the arteries following antihypertensive
      drug treatment   61
   Long-term drug treatment of hypertension in relation to the
      aging process   63

CHAPTER 7
Influence of Tobacco Consumption and Metabolic Abnormalities on Arterial Stiffness   **67**

Relationship of smoking and metabolic disorders to arterial stiffness   *67*
Metabolic disorders following drug therapy for hypertension   *69*
Atherosclerosis and increased arterial stiffness   *70*

CHAPTER 8
Conclusion: The Arterial System and the Therapeutic Trials of Hypertension   **73**

Basic assumptions of therapeutic trials and hypertensive large arteries: A critical review   *73*
Unanswered questions related to the role of the arteries in the treatment of hypertension   *79*

References   **83**
Index   **91**

1

INTRODUCTION

THE ARTERIAL SYSTEM AND THE
DEFINITION OF HYPERTENSION

Hypertension is the most important risk factor for cardiovascular morbid events affecting the brain, the heart, or the kidney. For that reason, the definition of hypertension has been largely popularized in experimental research and practical medicine. However, most of the morbid events due to hypertension are related to some alteration of the large arteries of the brain, the heart, or the kidney, such as ruptures, stenosis, or thrombosis. Despite this clinical evidence, the definition itself of hypertension has largely hampered the real importance of the status of the large arteries in this disease. It is the major point of this book to develop this basic assumption. For this, it is important to recognize that: (i) the definition of hypertension is arbitrary, (ii) an adequate definition of the disease should refer to a complete description of the blood pressure curve, and (iii) the lack of an adequate definition of hypertension tended to emphasize the role of small arteries and to neglect that of large arteries, thus creating a bias in the understanding of the clinical management and the pathophysiology of the disease.

THE ARBITRARY DEFINITION OF HYPERTENSION

In a given population, the distribution of blood pressure is gaussian and unimodal. When this distribution is considered, those persons with blood pressure above a certain arbitrary limit are said to have hypertension. This arbitrary limit is defined from two quantitative values determined from indirect brachial blood pressure measurements: peak-systolic blood pressure and end-diastolic blood pressure. Clearly, it is impossible to divide the population values into discrete categories on the basis of individual measurements. Nevertheless, from the clinical standpoint, a sharp distinction exists: a portion of the population (a minority) is defined as abnormal (hypertensive) and the remainder as normal (nor-

TABLE 1-1. *International classification of hypertension according to blood pressure (BP) level*

	SYSTOLIC BP (MM HG)		DIASTOLIC BP (MM HG)
Normotension	<140	and	<90
Mild hypertension	140–180	and/or	90–105
Subgroup: Borderline hypertension	140–160	and/or	90–95
Moderate and severe hypertension	>180	and/or	>105
Isolated systolic hypertension (ISH)	>160	and	<90
Subgroup: borderline ISH	140–160	and	<90

motensive) on the basis of blood pressure level. The usual criteria for the diagnosis of clinical hypertension are indicated in Table 1-1. Interestingly, this distinction does not depend on any qualitative intrinsic characteristics of the trait but exclusively on the fact that persons with higher pressure levels have a greater probability of having certain serious health problems (e.g., coronary heart disease, stroke, and renal failure).

As we mentioned above, for the diagnosis of hypertension, the two quantitative blood pressure values that are used are: peak-systolic blood pressure and end-diastolic blood pressure (Fig. 1-1, top). These two values are universally accepted, but it is important to realize that their use is no more than the consequence of their direct determination on the basis of a noninvasive technic at the site of the brachial artery. In fact, peak-systolic blood pressure and end-diastolic blood pressure are only two specific and arbitrary points of the blood pressure curve and do not give any information on the shape of the blood pressure curve itself. Nevertheless, *if the goal of research in hypertension is to define high blood pressure as a mechanical signal related to cardiovascular risk through alterations of the arterial wall, then the totality of the blood pressure curve should be studied in detail to define hypertension as a cardiovascular risk factor.*

FOURIER ANALYSIS OF THE BLOOD PRESSURE CURVE

To give a better description of the blood pressure curve, research workers in experimental hypertension defined, in addition to peak systolic and end-dias-

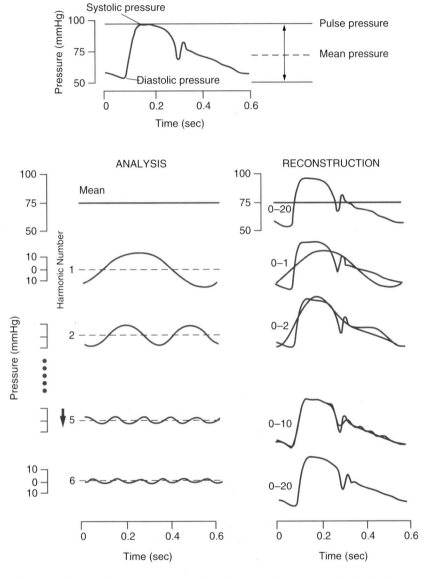

FIGURE 1-1. Blood pressure curve: pulsatile vs steady component. (See text.)

tolic blood pressure, another blood pressure value: mean arterial pressure. Mean arterial pressure is a virtual *steady* pressure, the area under the curve of which is equal to that of the pulsatile blood pressure curve recorded in living animals (Fig. 1-1, top). Although widely admitted, this definition minimizes one of the principal characteristics of the blood pressure curve in living animals and humans, that is, the presence of cyclic changes and hence of *pulsatility* of blood pressure. For this approach, Fourier analysis gives a better insight for a detailed description of the totality of the blood pressure curve.

Pressure and flow, especially in the larger arteries, are oscillatory. By relating only mean values of pressure and flow, as is usually done in a linear model of the circulation, the information contained in the waves shapes is lost. The use of Fourier analysis makes it possible to do both: the mean value of the wave is determined and its shape is described by a series of sine waves (harmonics) so that further mathematical analysis becomes possible[1].

The technique to derive a series of sine waves from a given pressure or flow signal is mathematically simple and unique, but the calculation, which is cumbersome, has been considerably improved the last years by digital computer. An example of Fourier analysis of the aortic pressure wave is given in Fig. 1-1. The harmonic zero reflects the mean value, which represents a sine wave with an infinite period. The first harmonic reflects the heart rate f, and higher harmonics have a frequency of $2f$, $3f$, and so forth. When all the sine waves are known, their addition leads to the mathematical reconstruction of the signal. As shown extensively by digital computers, in the cardiovascular system, about 20 harmonics are sufficient for an adequate reconstruction of the totality of the blood pressure curve.

Under that condition, a correct description of the curve does not only consider peak-systolic and end-diastolic blood pressure, but rather the mean pressure value and the oscillation around the mean (Fig. 1-1, top). Mean pressure (often calculated as diastolic pressure plus one-third pulse pressure) is related to steady flow, whereas the oscillation (often described as pulse pressure, the difference between systolic and diastolic pressure) is related to pulsatile flow.

The description in terms of mean pressure and pulse pressure may be considered as an oversimplification for the description of the totality of the blood pressure curve for several reasons. First, the variability of blood pressure is not taken into account. Second, in the arterial system, mean arterial pressure and pulse pressure are not completely independent variables: the higher the mean pressure, the higher the fluctuation around the mean.[1] However, it is a common finding in cardiovascular physiology that, for a given mean arterial pressure, different values of pulse pressure may be observed, either from one subject to another or in the same subjects when investigated beat by beat. This simple observation means that pulse pressure may be influenced by hemodynamic mechanisms different from that of mean arterial pressure and that these mechanisms may influence the shape of the blood pressure curve and therefore the definition of hypertension. This basic assumption will be detailed in the first section of this book.

THE DEFINITION OF HYPERTENSION ON THE
BASIS OF INCREASED MEAN ARTERIAL PRESSURE

In a linear model of the circulation, mean blood pressure represents the pressure drop *(delta P) obtained along a cylindrical tube in which a steady flow (Q) is obtained from a constant pump representing the heart.*[1] *There is a positive relationship between the pressure drop and flow, so that:*

$$delta\ P = R \times Q \qquad\qquad [1]$$

where R represents the opposition to flow (i.e., the slope of the relationship between delta P and Q and therefore, the totality of frictional forces that are opposed to flow).

Poiseuille was the first to show that, along the cylindrical tube, R was proportional to the viscosity v of the liquid and to the length l of the tube and inversely related to the radius r of the tube, according to the equation:

$$R = 8\ vl/3.14\ r^4 \qquad\qquad [2]$$

When this formula is applied to the totality of the arterial tree of living animals and men, it appears that if the length and the viscosity are considered as constant, the higher values of R are observed in the vessels with the lower radius, that is, in arterioles.

In this book, we do not wish to discuss the validity of the application of the Poiseuille law to the hemodynamics of the human vascular tree. However, we want to recall that because cardiac output is considered normal in hypertension and because hypertension may be defined as an increase in mean blood pressure (and therefore in *delta P*), hypertension is related to an increase in vascular resistance (R) and, therefore, to a reduction in the caliber and/or in the number of arterioles. This hemodynamic model is universally accepted for studies in experimental hypertension. In clinical hypertension, the situation is somewhat more complicated. Mean blood pressure (*MBP*) is often calculated from the empiric formula:

$$MBP = DBP + \tfrac{1}{3}\ PP$$

(*DBP* is diastolic blood pressure; *PP* is pulse pressure). Because pulse pressure is relatively low in comparison with MBP, MBP and *DBP* are often considered equivalent values to define hypertension in clinical practice. For that reason, in hypertension in humans, it is often believed that hypertension, evaluated from increased diastolic blood pressure (see Table 1-1), is due principally to an increase in vascular resistance. This is a very large approximation.

Younger   Older

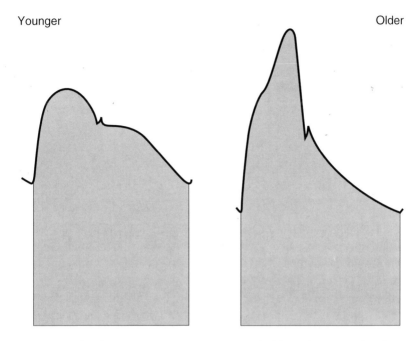

FIGURE 1-2. Blood pressure curve in younger and older subjects. Both subjects have the same cross-sectional area *(shaded area)* under the curve, and therefore the same mean arterial pressure. For the same mean arterial pressure, pulse pressure is higher in older than in younder subjects.

Although widely admitted, the assumption that hypertension (increased mean arterial pressure) is exclusively due to an increase in vascular resistance is untrue for several reasons. First, pulsatile pressure and pulsatile flow are not considered in this definition, which refers to a linear model. Second, for the same value of mean arterial pressure, several shapes of the blood pressure curve may be recorded, corresponding to quite different values of pulse pressure (Fig. 1-2). Finally, pulse pressure at any given value of ventricular ejection is known to be influenced by arterial changes, namely, arterial stiffness and the timing of reflected waves. Thus, through pulse-pressure regulation, the large arteries, in addition to the small arteries, may be considered as largely implicated in the definition of hypertensive vascular disease.

These observations are consistent with several epidemiologic and therapeutic findings well established in the field of clinical hypertension. Investigators have focused primarily on the role played by mean arterial pressure in alterations of the vascular system during chronic hypertension. Mean arterial pressure (often approximated from diastolic blood pressure) per se has been assumed to play a determinant role in alterations of vascular structure and function among a variety of determinants, including neural factors, humoral agents, and genetic factors. However, the evidence has not been entirely convincing, because the degree of reversal of arteriolar changes during treatment of chronic hypertension has not often matched the degree of reduction in mean or diastolic arterial pressure. Some epidemiologic and experimental studies[1,2] have raised the possibility that pulse pressure may be a determinant of vascular structure and function. Thus, when evaluating the effects of mechanical stress on the arterial system, it is necessary not only to take into account steady (i.e., mean) parameters but also to consider pulsatile parameters.

THE ARTERIES AS AN IMPORTANT BIAS IN THE RESEARCH OF HYPERTENSION

Because large arteries were neglected in the hemodynamic definition of hypertension, several aspects of the pathophysiology of the disease have been largely dismissed in experimental hypertension. On the one hand, the disease in animals is exclusively defined by the level of mean arterial pressure and vascular resistance and constriction of arterioles. On the other hand, because the animal models have no definite relevance in terms of cardiovascular morbidity and mortality, the large arteries are not considered as having a specific part in the mechanisms of hypertension. Finally, for simple methodological reasons mainly related to the size of the vascular tissue, the cellular aspects of the hypertensive disease in animals are principally studied at the site of the large arteries, mainly the aorta. Nevertheless, the deduced pathophysiological mechanisms are generally applied to the resistant arteries (i.e., the arterioles) and then integrated as a factor that plays a role in the disturbance of the blood pressure regulation observed in hypertension. This widely used approach in animal hypertension is particularly confusing because aortic changes are exclusively related to the buffering function of large arteries and, therefore, to the pulse pressure regulation. In contrast, arteriolar changes point to some abnormality of the resistant function and, therefore, to mean arterial pressure regulation. Thus, the investigations of the cellular aspects of hypertension on large arteries are not relevant when exploring the resistant function of arterioles. One of the purposes of this book is to explain that this mismatch, which has been popularized by numerous studies in experimental hypertension, are easily resolved when two important characteristics of hypertensive cardiovascular disease are recognized, namely, that (i) large arteries define the exact site in which blood pressure is measured both in clinical and experimental hypertension, and (ii) large arteries figure directly in the definition and in the pathophysiology of the hypertensive vascular disease.

Finally, the general purpose of this book is three-fold: (i) to analyze the physiological connections between the function of large arteries and the blood pressure regulation, (ii) to investigate the particularities of the arterial system

in hypertension, and (iii) to apply the described pathophysiological mechanisms to the study of the response of the arterial system to antihypertensive
drug therapy. Most of these findings relate exclusively to human hypertension.
Experimental studies are analyzed only in their direct relationship with clinical data.

SECTION

I

ARTERIES IN UNTREATED CLINICAL HYPERTENSION

2

THE ARTERIAL SYSTEM

SIMPLIFIED BASIC CONCEPTS

In this chapter, some of the more useful physiological aspects of arterial hemo-dynamics in the area of clinical hypertension are summarized, almost exactly as they are described by Nichols and O'Rourke.[1]

THE FUNCTION OF ARTERIES

The arterial system has two distinct functions: (i) arteries as conduits by means of which an adequate supply of blood is delivered to body tissues; and (ii) arteries as cushions whereby the pulsations resulting from intermittent ventricular ejection are dampened. These functions are interrelated.

Arteries as Conduits

As conduits, the arteries have the role of carrying an adequate supply of blood from the heart to the peripheral organs and tissues of the body. A continuous, steady, and constant flow of blood is required for metabolic activity. To maintain this flow, there must be a steady head of pressure that will overcome the energy losses resulting from the viscosity of the blood and friction; that is, to overcome vascular resistance (see Chapter 1). Vascular resistance is defined by the relationship between steady or mean blood pressure and blood flow. Mean blood pressure is calculated by measuring the area under the blood pressure curve and then dividing this measurement by the time interval involved (Figs. 1-1 and 1-2). Mean blood pressure is determined by cardiac output and vascular resistance. The efficiency of the arterial conduit function depends on the arterial caliber and the constancy of mean blood pressure, with an almost imperceptible mean pressure gradient between the ascending aorta and the peripheral arteries.

Arteries as Cushions

The chief role of arteries as cushions is to smooth out the pressure oscillations resulting from intermittent ventricular ejection. Hemodynamically, pulsatile flow and pulsatile pressure characterize the cushioning function. Large arteries can instantaneously accommodate the volume of blood ejected from the ventricles, storing part of the stroke volume during systole and draining this volume during diastole, thus permitting continuous perfusion of peripheral organs and tissues. The cushioning function is due to the viscoelastic properties of the arterial walls and can be evaluated in two ways: (i) the "Windkessel," or air chamber effect (time domain), and (ii) wave propagation (frequency domain).

In the Windkessel model it is important that the reader recall that, on the one hand, during systole, the pressure rise up to the time of peak velocity depends on left ventricular performance and on the distensibility of the ascending aorta. Thus, the more rigid the arterial wall, the greater the peak systolic pressure. On the other hand, after closure of the aortic valve, arterial pressure gradually falls as blood drains into the peripheral vessels. The rate of the fall in pressure and the duration of the diastolic time interval determine the minimum diastolic pressure. The rate at which the pressure falls is influenced by the rate of outflow, that is, peripheral resistance, and by arterial viscoelasticity. At a given vascular resistance, the drop in diastolic pressure will be greater if the stiffness of large arteries is augmented.

Arterial wall viscoelasticity is also a determining element of the speed of wave propagation (pulse-wave velocity) and of the timing of wave reflections. Stiffening of the arteries increases pulse-wave velocity and may cause an earlier return of the reflected wave. This superimposition on an incident pressure wave serves to increase pulse and systolic pressure further. Other mechanisms may also contribute to early return of reflected waves as reflection sites closer to the heart and also change reflection coefficients. These mechanisms, detailed in Chapter 3, have a great influence on the systolic peak level.

Finally, the efficiency of arteries as cushions depends on the compliance and distensibility of arterial walls and on the viscoelastic properties of the vessels. The disturbance in the cushioning function has a deleterious effect on the heart upstream, due to the inadequate increase in systolic pressure and the relative decrease in aortic diastolic pressure at any given mean arterial pressure value. These arterial pressure changes, which are described below, are the following: the mismatch between aortic impedance and ventricular ejection; increased pulsatile energy losses in arteries; increased ventricular oxygen consumption; increased ventricular afterload and left ventricular hypertrophy; and compromised coronary perfusion.

Arterial Changes and Blood Pressure Regulation

As a result of the conduit and cushioning functions of arteries and in accordance with Fourier analysis of the blood pressure curve, arterial pressure has two components that reflect the influence of various hemodynamic factors (see Fig. 1-1): (i) mean blood pressure and (ii) the pulsatile component. Mean blood pressure is determined by cardiac output and vascular resistance, which are in turn determined by the caliber and number of the small arteries and arterioles. Pulse pressure—the pulsatile component—represents the oscillation around the mean pressure, the systole and diastole being the highs and lows of the oscillation. The magnitude of the pulse pressure is determined by the pattern of left ventricular ejection, the viscoelastic and propagative properties of large arteries, and the timing of the reflected waves. These two components of blood pressure have a marked effect on the viscoelastic and propagative properties of the arterial system.

The distinction between the two functions is particularly important when we consider high blood pressure[2] (see Fig. 2-1). Whereas an increase in vascular resistance causes a proportionate rise in systolic and diastolic pressure (and therefore mean arterial pressure), a reduction in the viscoelasticity of the arterial wall only modifies the shape of the curve, with systolic and diastolic pressures increasing and decreasing, respectively, without change in the value of mean arterial pressure (see Fig. 2-1). These patterns have a direct relation to the hemodynamics of hypertension in the middle-aged (increase in vascular resistance) and in the elderly (decrease in arterial compliance).

THE PRESSURE-VOLUME RELATIONSHIP

The capability of the aorta and large arteries to instantaneously accommodate left ventricular stroke volume depends on the pressure-volume relationship in a given artery. The positive pressure-volume relationship thus obtained oversimplifies the stress-strain relationship that defines conceptually the mechanical properties of the arteries. Stress is defined as $P \times r/h$, P being the transmural pressure, r and h the radius and thickness of the artery, respectively. Strain is defined as $\Delta l/l$, where l is the length of the material at baseline and Δl the change in length for a given stress. The stress-strain relationship is discussed in greater detail in the Appendix to this chapter. For the study of the pressure-volume relationship, the r/h ratio is considered of little significance by comparison with P. However, $\Delta l/l$ is replaced in a cylindric artery by $\Delta V/V$, that is, the change in volume (ΔV) from baseline volume (V). Because, in a cylindric artery, the length of the artery may be considered as constant, the pressure-diameter relationship is often used instead of the pressure-volume relationship

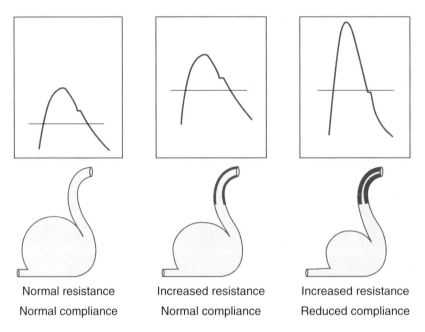

Normal resistance   Increased resistance   Increased resistance
Normal compliance   Normal compliance   Reduced compliance

FIGURE 2-1. Effects of increased vascular resistance and reduced arterial compliance on the blood pressure curve, particularly on peak systolic and end-diastolic pressure valves. The *straight horizontal line* represents mean arterial pressure.

to describe the mechanical properties of the arteries. For an understanding of the pressure-volume relationship, capacitance, compliance, and unstressed volume must be defined.

Capacitance

Capacitance is the relation of the contained volume of the arteries (total vasculature or segmental arteries) to a given transmural pressure over the physiological range of pressure. Capacitance is influenced by the viscoelasticity of the vessels—the compliance—and the "geometry" of the vasculature—the unstressed volume (Fig. 2-2).

Compliance

Compliance is the change in dimension (ΔV) following a change in stress (ΔP). In physiology, compliance is defined as the change in volume (ΔV) divided by the change in pressure (ΔP), that is, $C = \Delta V/\Delta P$ (see Fig. 2-2). Compliance represents the slope of the pressure-volume relationship at a specific point of the

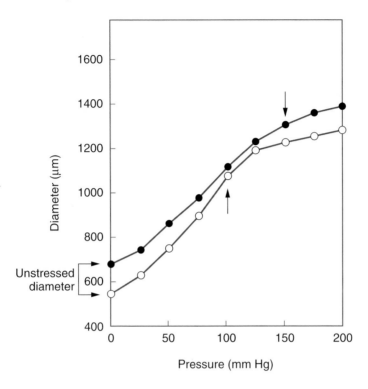

FIGURE 2-2. Pressure-diameter (volume) relationship in a given artery: the slope at a given pressure defines compliance in normotensive *(open circles)* and hypertensive *(filled circles)* rats. *Arrows* indicate the operating pressure in each group. (From Caputo L, et al. *J Hypertension* 1992; 10 (suppl 6): 527–530.)

pressure-volume curve, which is not linear. Indeed, the tunica media of the arteries is responsible for its physical properties. The arterial media consists of smooth muscle cells and connective tissue containing elastin and collagen. The pressure-volume relationship is therefore nonlinear. The elastin fibers assume the tension at low distending pressures, whereas at high distending pressures tension is borne by the collagen fibers, which are less distensible, and the arterial wall becomes less compliant. Compliance can only be defined in terms of a given pressure. Subsequently, compliance depends predominantly on the intrinsic elasticity and amount of material that makes up the wall of the artery and less on the level of blood pressure.

Unstressed Volume

Unstressed volume is the volume of blood (or the diameter) for a given vessel at zero transmural pressure (see Fig. 2-2). A vessel's capacitance depends not only on the $\Delta V/\Delta P$ but also on the initial volume. For the same compliance, the vascular system with greater unstressed volume has greater capacitance. Even with a reduced compliance, the vascular system with a higher unstressed volume may have a maintained or even enhanced capacitance (see Fig. 2-2). Comparisons of the viscoelastic properties of structures with different initial dimensions and volumes may be facilitated by expressing compliance relative to the initial volume as a coefficient of volume distensibility: $\Delta V/\Delta P \cdot V$, where $\Delta V/\Delta P$ is compliance and V is baseline volume.

Arterial volume per unit length is equal to arterial cross-sectional area, depending on arterial diameter (D). Thus compliance is also determined from the pressure-diameter relationship as $C = \Delta D/\Delta P$; the volume distensibility is expressed as $\Delta D/\Delta P \cdot D$. The reciprocal of volume distensibility may be expressed as the Peterson elastic modulus E_p (wall pressure for 100% diameter increase) ($E_p = \Delta P \cdot D/\Delta D$), or as Young's modulus E (wall tension per centimeter wall thickness for 100% diameter increase) ($E = \Delta P \cdot D/h \cdot \Delta D$), where ΔP and ΔD are changes in pressure and diameter, respectively, about a mean diameter (D) in an artery with wall thickness h.[1,3] Since Young's modulus involves arterial thickness, it represents the slope of the stress-strain relationship. It is considered to be the most accurate index for the evaluation of arterial rigidity (see Appendix), but arterial thickness in most cases is difficult to evaluate, particularly in humans, and therefore in recent years compliance and distensibility have been the most widely used parameters.[1,3,4]

GEOMETRY VERSUS MECHANICS

The relationship between the geometric characteristics of arteries (diameter) and the mechanical properties of arterial walls (compliance) at a given blood pressure is complex. As shown in many animal experiments,[1,3–5] problems are encountered with three different characteristics: (i) the nonlinear elastic behavior of the arterial wall, (ii) the specific effects of smooth muscle contraction on the stiffness and diameter of the arteries, and (iii) the direct effect of pressure changes on arterial diameter. The relationship between diameter and compliance complicates the analysis of changes in compliance under various physiological conditions or following administration of vasoactive drugs. Alterations in diameter and compliance could be the result of changes in blood pressure or of the direct action of vasoactive agents or physiological stimuli on the arterial walls, principally on the smooth muscle cells.[3]

Under normal conditions and with blood pressure held at a constant level, arterial compliance in vitro is reduced as the artery is dilated.[3] This hemodynamic pattern results directly from an increase in wall tension as the diameter increases and to the transfer of this tension from elastin to the less extensible collagen fibers. The situation is more complex in vivo because capacitance may be increased by an increase in diameter, that is, by vasodilation, or by a reduction in tension on the arterial walls, that is, by relaxation of smooth muscle cells even without geometric change. It has been shown that vasoactive drugs, including calcium channel blockers, nitrates, and angiotensin converting enzyme inhibitors, dilate medium-sized arteries in parallel with an increase in compliance.[6] This paradoxical finding is explained on the basis of alignment of arterial smooth muscle in series with collagen fibers and in parallel with elastic fibers. The result of the relaxation in arterial smooth muscle is transfer of wall stress from collagenous elements to elastin fibers[1].

Another major question with regard to the action of vasoactive drugs on arteries is whether the relaxation of arterial smooth muscle is due to an in situ effect or whether it may also be the result of arteriolar dilation or a combination of both. Any change in blood flow velocity at the site of a large artery may cause a change in arterial diameter via the mechanism of flow dilation.[7] This mechanism, which has been demonstrated not only experimentally but also in hypertensive and normotensive humans,[8] has two important features: (i) the change in blood flow velocity may be mediated downstream by a change in arterial diameter, and (ii) the increased velocity, and thus the increase in shear stress, causes an increase in arterial diameter through a mechanism that involves the release of relaxing and constrictive factors of the endothelium.[7] Some aspects of this important mechanism are detailed in Section II of this book.

APPENDIX
THE STRESS-STRAIN RELATIONSHIP

Pressurizing a vessel distends the wall in the circumferential and longitudinal directions and simultaneously narrows the wall thickness. The circumferential and longitudinal stresses are tensile and the radial stress that narrows the wall thickness is compressive. Only the circumferential stress[1-5] will be detailed here.

Circumferential stress is comparable to the wall tension (force) given by the law of Laplace but accounts for the finite wall thickness of arteries. Indeed, the law of Laplace states that the tension (T, force per unit length) in the wall of a very thin cylindrical shell is related to transmural pressure (PT) and radius (r); as $T = PT \times r$. The circumferential stress on the wall depends on the wall thickness, however.

The circumferential distending force ($F_{\theta D}$) for a thin-wall is the product of the transmural pressure and the area over which that distending transmural pressure is exerted or

$$F_{\theta D} = PT \times d_i \times l \qquad [1]$$

where *PT* is transmural pressure, d_i is internal diameter, and *l* is vessel length. Deformation of an elastic or viscoelastic material elicits a retractive force ($F_{\Theta R}$), which is the product of the wall stress in the circumferential direction and the area over which that stress is exerted, or

$$F_{\Theta R} = \sigma\Theta \times h \times l \qquad [2]$$

where $\sigma\Theta$ is circumferential stress exerted by the tissue and *h* is wall thickness. Because distending and retracting forces are equal ($F_{\Theta D} = F_{\Theta R}$) at equilibrium, Equations [1] and [2] may be set equal and solved algebraically for $\sigma\Theta$. The mean $\sigma\Theta$ is then

$$\sigma\Theta = PT \times r_i/h \qquad [3]$$

where r_i is internal radius.

Circumferential stress may be used to compute strain–stress relations and incremental elastic moduli to assess the elastic properties of the arteries. This has mainly been done in vitro, with steady increases in distending pressure.[1,3–5] Provided arterial wall motion is detected during each cardiac cycle, the in vivo strain–stress relation to the artery may be computed. In vivo arterial wall motion occurs predominantly in the circumferential direction; much smaller changes occur in the longitudinal direction. The shape of the diameter oscillations closely resembles the form of the pressure pulse. Extrathoracic systemic arteries change 8%–10% in diameter with each cardiac cycle, whereas the diameter of the intrathoracic arteries changes 8%–18% with each cardiac cycle.[1] The circumferential strain ($\Sigma\Theta$) is

$$\Sigma\Theta = (d - d_o)/d_o \qquad [4]$$

where *d* is the observed diameter and d_o is the original diameter. Variously, d_o has been defined either as the diameter of the retracted, totally unloaded vessel, as diameter at low or 0 mm Hg pressure, or as unstressed diameter.[1–3] For materials having linear strain–stress relations, the ratio of stress to strain may be used to compute Young's modulus of elasticity: the stretching force per unit cross-sectional area required to elongate a strip of a vessel wall by 100%. However, for materials with nonlinear strain–stress relations, the slope of the strain–stress curve may be used to compute an incremental elastic modulus, defined, for a cylindrical vessel with wall stiffness that are equal in all directions, as:

$$E_{inc} = \sigma\Theta \times 0.75/\Sigma\Theta \qquad [5]$$

In in vitro preparations, the stress–strain relationship is determined using the distending pressure and, at each level of distending pressure, the internal radius of the vessel and the wall thickness. Stress is calculated following Equation [3] and strain—the fractional increase in circumferential length—following Equation [4].

3

PULSATILE PRESSURE AND HYPERTENSION IN LARGE ARTERIES

It has been recognized in recent years that increases in pulsatile pressure and wave reflections in hypertension should be studied in connection with the arterial changes observed in this disease.

THE PULSATILE COMPONENT

Invasive hemodynamic studies in the thoracic aorta[1] and indirect measurements of brachial artery pulse pressure in humans have brought about the recognition of the increase in pulse pressure in hypertension. The major contribution of arterial pulsatile hemodynamic studies in this field has been the demonstration that whereas mean arterial pressure is poorly modified along the arterial system, the pulse pressure increases from centrally to peripherally due to several factors: (i) the progressive decrease in arterial cross-sectional area; (ii) the progressive increase in arterial rigidity; and (iii), most important, the summation of wave reflections along the arterial tree. These changes have been poorly studied in clinical hypertension because of the difficulty in determining pulse pressure in vivo in arterial segments using noninvasive methods.

Noninvasive Methods of Measurement

The accuracy of recording noninvasively the blood pressure wave contour along the arterial tree has been improved by the technique of applanation (flattening) tonometry. This technique employs a pencil-type probe incorporating a high-fidelity strain gauge transducer[9,10] (Millar Instruments, Inc., Houston). It is well known that applanation of a curved surface of a pressure-containing structure under the sensor allows direct measurement of the pressure within the structure (Fig. 3-1). The accuracy of this method was tested on the exposed femoral artery of the dog and on the radial and carotid arteries of humans percutaneously.[9,10]

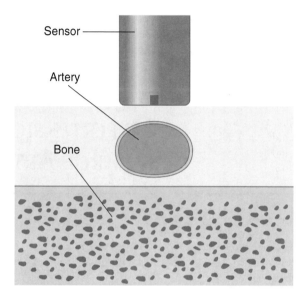

FIGURE 3-1. Principle of applanation tonometry.[9]

The waveforms recorded in dogs were virtually identical to direct intra-arterials recordings. Fourier analysis showed a highly significant correlation between direct and indirect recordings. In humans who underwent catheterization, blood pressure was measured at the same time by two methods: (i) invasively, at the site of the aortic arch; and (ii) noninvasively, at the site of the common carotid. A significant positive correlation ($r = .92$) was observed[11] with a slope equal to 1.05 and an intercept that was not significantly different from zero (0.4 mm Hg). Another study measured brachial artery pulse pressure by conventional sphygmomanometry and radial artery pulse pressure by applanation tonometry. The two were strongly correlated: $r = .97$; slope: 98; intercept: 1.4 mm Hg.[12]

 The positioning of the transducer over the site of the artery is important for clinical investigation[9–12] because the transducer is small relative to arterial size and artifacts may be caused by movements of the operator's hand or of the subject. Movements can be avoided by fixing the probe using a stereotaxic instrument. The operator should, of course, be relaxed and comfortable. The hold-down force should be adequate to achieve accurate applanation, taking care to avoid excessive force so as to prevent distortion of the diastolic component of the wave shape. Also, the probe should be held as close to perpendicular as possible to the axis of the vessel. An adequate evaluation requires three to four weeks. With this procedure variability of measurements between observers and by the same observer is less than 10%.[9–12]

TABLE 3-1. *Analysis of carotid pulse wave characteristics in control subjects and in patients with end-stage renal disease (ESRD)[12,22]*

	CONTROL SUBJECTS	ESRD PATIENTS
Radial artery *PP* (mm Hg)	60.7 ± 16.1	73.7 ± 22.0***
Carotid artery *PP* (mm Hg)	57.3 ± 19.6	73.2 ± 25.7***
Carotid *PP*/Radial *PP* (ratio)	0.93 ± 0.14	0.99 ± 0.15*
Augmentation index (mm Hg)	7.5 ± 10.5	19.0 ± 15.2***
Augmentation index (%)	9.8 ± 15.6	23.2 ± 15.0***
Heart period (ms)	909 ± 149	840 ± 145**
Aortic *PWV* (cm/s)	930 ± 196	1035 ± 238**

[a]For the interpretation, see text and Fig. 3-5.
Values are mean ± standard deviation.
PP, pulse pressure; *PWV*, pulse wave velocity.
*$p < 0.02$; **$p < 0.01$; ***$p < 0.001$.

Characteristics of Pulse Pressure

Pulse pressure measurements have been carried out noninvasively in subjects with essential hypertension and in those with end-stage renal disease. The results differ greatly according to age.[11-13]

In younger subjects (defined as those less than 50 years of age), pulse pressure increases significantly from the central to the peripheral arteries, principally because of an increase in systolic pressure and additionally to a modest decrease in diastolic blood pressure. Carotid artery pressure, which is virtually identical to aortic pulse pressure, is lower than radial and femoral artery pulse pressures (Table 3-1 and Fig. 3-2). The highest pressure values are seen in the common femoral artery (see Fig. 3-2). Although absolute values are higher in the hypertensive group, the pulse pressure gradient along the arterial tree is similar in both normotensive and hypertensive subjects. In rats, in contrast, the gradient seen in the normotensive animals is not observed in the hypertensive animals,[14] probably because of the short body height of rats. This aspect is discussed further below.

In older subjects (those above 50 years of age), pulse pressure is similar throughout the arterial system. This pattern is due to the fact that carotid artery pulse pressure increases markedly with age, but femoral pressure does not.[11] This modification with age is due to the high wave velocity, the result of which is that pressure oscillations become almost synchronous everywhere in the arterial tree[1]. This picture is observed in both older normotensive and older hypertensive subjects, particularly in systolic hypertension, and in those patients with hypertension and end-stage renal disease.[6,11-13]

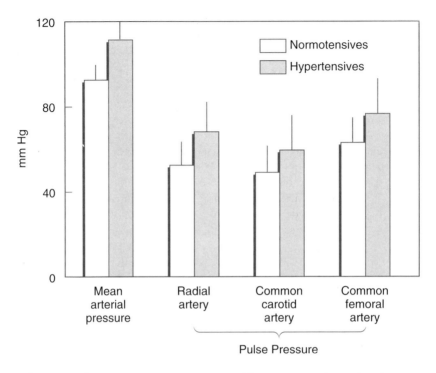

FIGURE 3-2. Pulse pressure in normotensive and hypertensive subjects less than 50 years of age (personal data).

An indirect evaluation of pulse pressure transmission along the arterial tree of humans is provided by Doppler studies to determine the ratio between ankle and brachial systolic blood pressure. This ratio ranges from 101% to 120% in younger subjects and approaches 100% in older subjects, whether they be normotensive or hypertensive.[15]

Epidemiologic Aspects

Epidemiologic studies have found a close correlation between blood pressure level and the incidence of cardiovascular diseases.[16] The particular roles of systolic and diastolic pressure have also been investigated.[16] It has been recognized that diastolic and mean blood pressures are more strongly related to cardiovascular risk before age 45 years, whereas systolic pressure is more strongly related to cardiovascular disease after age 45.[17] In these studies, however, only systolic, diastolic, and mean blood pressures were taken into account. The role of the pulsatile component, independent of mean arterial blood pressure, in cardiovascular morbidity and mortality was not evaluated.

The relationship between blood pressure—mean arterial pressure and pulse pressure—and cardiovascular risk was investigated in 18,336 men and 9351 women living in Paris, and ranging in age from 40 to 69 years.[18] Because mean arterial pressure and pulse pressure are closely interrelated, the investigators used a principal component analysis to define two independent parameters that reflected, independently, the steady component (mean pressure) and pulsatile components (pulse pressure). The findings from this cross-sectional analysis that were related to the steady component were similar to those reported earlier for diastolic or mean blood pressure in most published epidemiologic studies, that is, the level of mean or diastolic blood pressure is a strong determinant of the risk of stroke, coronary heart disease, and kidney disease.[16,17] In contrast, the pulsatile component was related exclusively to cardiac changes, as judged on the basis of electrocardiographic indices of ventricular hypertrophy. The specific role of pulsatile pressure as a cardiovascular risk factor was confirmed by a 10-year survival analysis.[18] In women over 55 years of age, particularly, this index correlated independently with coronary mortality and not with cerebrovascular death.

On the basis of pulsatile arterial hemodynamics,[1,2] the role of pulse pressure as an independent cardiovascular risk factor is easy to understand. An increase in pulse pressure is common in people over 50 years of age as a result of increased aortic stiffening. An increase in aortic stiffening causes an increase in systolic pressure and a decrease in diastolic pressure at any given value of mean arterial pressure. The increase in systole is responsible for a disproportionate increase in end-systole stress. This is the principal factor in the development of ventricular hypertrophy. In hypertensive subjects, cardiac mass has been shown to be strongly associated with carotid pulse pressure, independently of the level of mean arterial pressure[12,19] (Fig. 3-3). The decrease in diastolic pressure caused by aortic stiffening may have adverse effects on coronary perfusion.[1,2] The coronary circulation is the only circulation in the arterial system in which perfusion pressure is diastolic pressure, which is influenced by both vascular resistance and aortic compliance. In contrast, the perfusion pressure of all the other regional circulations is mean arterial pressure, which is influenced exclusively by vascular resistance.

WAVE REFLECTIONS AND HYPERTENSION

General Concepts

On the basis of pulsatile hemodynamic studies, it is well established that the factors influencing pulse pressure may be analyzed as the summation of an incident pressure wave originating from the heart and a reflected wave returning to the heart from the resistant vessels in the peripheral circulation (Fig. 3-4). The for-

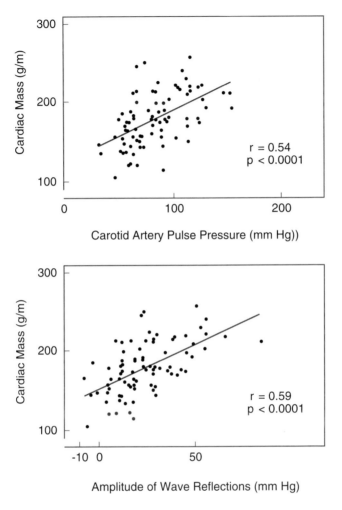

FIGURE 3-3. Above, the relationship between carotid pulse pressure and cardiac mass. Below, the relationship between the amplitude of wave reflections (see Fig. 3-5) and cardiac mass in a hypertensive population with end-stage renal disease.[24]

ward wave is simply influenced by ventricular ejection and stiffening of the aorta. On the other hand, the backward reflected wave depends on (1) the value of reflection coefficients, (2) stiffening of the arteries, and (3) the most important parameter, the site of reflection points.[1] For given values of reflection coefficients, increased pulse wave velocity and reflection sites closer to the heart produce a more pronounced aortic backward wave, with a more substantial summation of forward and backward waves, higher pulse pressure, and higher systolic peak.

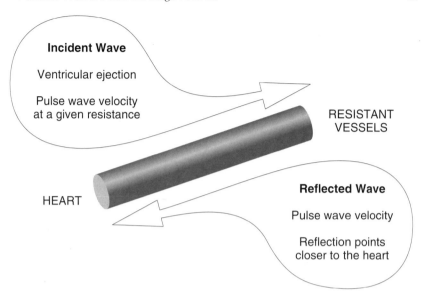

FIGURE 3-4. The pulse pressure curve as the mathematical summation between an incident and a reflected pressure wave.[1]

Normally, pulse wave velocity is relatively low and reflection points are principally observed at the early narrowing of small resistant vessels, causing a return of reflection waves during diastole. As shown in younger subjects in Figure 1-2, this aspect reflects a favorable condition, contributing to maintenance of mean arterial pressure and to adequate coupling between the vessels and the heart. With aging and high blood pressure, however, pulse wave velocity increases markedly and additional reflecting waves operate closer to the heart, causing a return of reflected waves during the systolic component and the appearance of a late systolic peak[1,20] (Figs. 3-4 and 3-5). This promotes a disproportionate increase in systolic over diastolic pressure and a mismatch between heart and vessels.

Increased pulse wave velocity is a classic finding in hypertension.[1] The role of reflection points closer to the heart over diastolic blood pressure is more difficult to demonstrate. It results from the finding of a disproportionate increase in systolic pressure in specific populations, e.g., patients with coarctation of the aorta[1] or with traumatic amputation of the lower limbs.[21] In both populations, reflection points closer to the heart are related to the coarctation or amputation of arterial segments that are closer to the heart by comparison with physiological reflection sites. Recently, it was noted that increased wave reflections in the aorta are particularly observed in subjects with low body height. In these subjects, the reduced length of the vasculature favors reflection

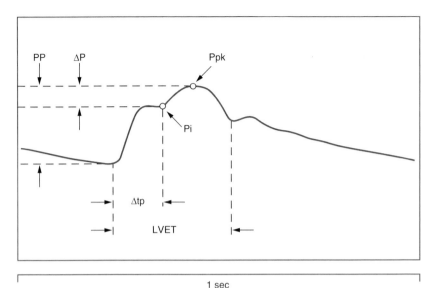

Figure 3-5. Carotid pulse-pressure waveform.[22] LVET, left ventricular ejection time. (See text for abbreviations.)

sites nearer the heart and therefore higher systolic peak values.[13,22] Similar patterns are seen in rats; the aortic pulse pressure gradient observed in normotensive rats is not present in hypertensive rats.[14]

   In hypertensive subjects, invasive evaluation techniques for determination of the aortic impedance spectrum have been used to quantify wave reflections for many years.[1] Recently, noninvasive techniques have become available.

Noninvasive Evaluation

In evaluating wave reflections, it is important to recall that aortic and carotid artery pulse pressure (*PP*) waveforms in humans are similar.[1,23] Therefore, they may be easily recognized on the carotid pressure waveform obtained by applanation tonometry. As detailed by Murgo et al.,[23] the pressure curve generally manifests an inflection point (P_i) that divides the pressure wave into an early and mid-to-late systolic peak (see Fig. 3-5). This peak (P_{pk}) is due to the reflected wave returning from peripheral site(s) causing an increase in pulse and systolic blood pressure.[22,23] It is quantified as $\Delta P/PP(\Delta P = P_{pk} - P_i)$. The time from the foot of the pressure wave to the foot of the late systolic peak (Δt_p) has been considered to be the travel time of the pulse wave to a peripheral reflecting site(s) and its return.[1,23] Study of the relationship between the aortic pressure waveform and aortic input impedance has shown that a larger secondary rise of

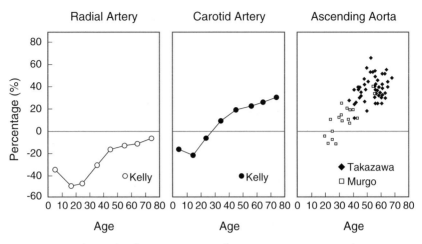

FIGURE 3-6. Relationship between wave reflections (percentage) and age in nor-motensive subjects. Note that wave reflections increase more markedly with age in the ascending aorta. (Kelly, Takazawa, and Murgo data reported in reference 9.)

PP is associated with an enhanced oscillatory impedance spectrum caused by differences in the magnitude of wave reflections or inflection interaction for different sites, or a combination of these.[1,23] Table 3-1 and Figure 3-3 provided examples for noninvasive study of wave reflections. Figure 3-3 indicates that the amplitude of wave reflections $(P_{pk} - P_i)$ is strongly associated with increased cardiac mass in hypertensive subjects.[24]

Quantification of Wave Reflections

Noninvasive studies of wave reflections have documented the age-associated increase in late systolic peak.[1,9,23] The results of these studies indicate that wave reflections in the thoracic aorta increase markedly with age, much more so than in the peripheral arteries (Fig. 3-6). This mechanism is amplified in people with hypertension, in whom, at any age, wave reflections are more important than in those with normal blood pressure.[13,22] Table 3-1 showed that wave reflections are significantly increased in hypertensive subjects with end-stage renal disease.[22] The same increases are found in middle-aged subjects with essential hypertension and in elderly subjects, to a greater extent, with systolic hypertension.[1,13] In all subjects, wave reflections return very early, that is, they return in the systolic part of the blood pressure curve, thereby causing a high systolic peak (see Fig. 1-2). Finally, owing to the age-related increase in aortic wave reflections and to their faster increase in high blood pressure, pulse pressure in hypertension becomes identical throughout the arterial tree in persons over 50 years of age. This changing pattern in wave reflections with age explains why carotid pulse pressure (and not femoral pulse pressure) increases markedly with age (see p. 23).[11]

Importance of Wave Reflections in Clinical Hypertension

In subjects with hypertension, because of the increase in mean arterial pressure and pulse-wave velocity and reflection sites closer to the heart, reflected waves are altered and mostly return during systole. This has two exacerbating effects: (1) mean diastolic pressure tends to decrease, resulting in a decrease in coronary perfusion;[1,2] (2) the late systolic peak increases significantly and, through the increase in end-systolic stress, promotes cardiac hypertrophy. Of interest, in humans with hypertension, aortic stiffening and mostly increased aortic wave reflections are strongly associated with left ventricular hypertrophy, especially in those with end-stage renal disease[6,12,24] (see Fig. 3-3).

One major point to note here is that altered wave reflections may be reversed by vasodilator therapy. This has been demonstrated by the administration of nitrates. This important aspect has been developed by O'Rourke's group and others.[25–28]

With administration of nitrates, later reflection waves may be obtained even without pulse-wave velocity changes, because the distance between the heart and the reflection points is increased by the effect of the drug. As early as 1964, Taylor[29] demonstrated that an increase in arterial cross section at the bifurcations of peripheral arteries could, in theory, produce this type of change in reflection patterns. These geometrical changes might reduce the intensity of reflections at the bifurcations so that the total reflections would begin more exclusively at vascular terminations. The resultant delayed wave reflections would help to decrease considerably aortic systolic and pulse pressure.[25,26] This mechanism operates with nitrates by reducing the amplitude of peripheral vascular reflections and delaying their return to the aortic root without substantially changing ventricular ejection and vascular resistance.[25,26] In addition, administration of nitrates results in a greater dilation of peripheral arteries than of the thoracic aorta.[27,28] This finding agrees with the model described by Taylor.[29]

4

CROSS-SECTIONAL AREA, STIFFNESS, AND THICKNESS OF THE LARGE ARTERIES IN HYPERTENSION

This chapter summarizes recent knowledge on the diameter, stiffness, and thickness of the large arteries in hypertension.

CROSS-SECTIONAL AREA AND DIAMETER CHANGES

Until recently, changes in the cross-sectional area of large arteries have been poorly studied in laboratory animals because of the lack of adequate methodology. Most findings in this area have come from clinical investigations in humans.

Echo-Doppler Evaluations

Echocardiographic and pulse Doppler velocimetric methods developed over recent decades have provided noninvasive ways to determine the caliber of large arteries, that is, the central aorta, brachial, and the common carotid and femoral arteries.[30,31] Although resolution was poor in early studies, recently devices have been described that measure arterial diameter and wall motion transcutaneously by tracking signals from both the anterior and posterior walls. Earlier methods produced superimposed echo signals from the tissue surrounding the artery and this, together with poor alignment of the ultrasonic beam, resulted in major changes in the echo waveform amplitude.[32–35] The newer instruments have adequate linearity, dynamic range, and tracking speed, even when the ratio of signal to noise is not high. In the following paragraphs, we summarize previously published information on methodological aspects in clinical hypertension.

Today, innovative procedures are used to measure vessel wall displacements of the peripheral arteries. The Walltrack system[32] was developed to measure the wall motion of large arteries (e.g., brachial, common carotid) after localization by echocardiography. With accurate determination of Doppler frequency (phase-locked echo tracking), no stereotaxic apparatus is needed. The Diarad system[33] is used to obtain the pressure-diameter curve of the radial artery by coupling measurement of variations in arterial diameter to readings of digital blood pressure. This system uses two techniques: (i) a pulsed Doppler system coupled to the echo-tracking system facilitates localization of the radial artery; (ii) a 10-MHz transducer and an 11-mm focal length provide high spatial resolution and excellent reproducibility for measuring internal diameter and pulsatile changes of the artery provided the probe is fixed stereotaxically. The methodology has been described in detail for both devices[28,32,33,36] and is summarized below.

The Walltrack system measures time-dependent changes in diameter of the artery relative to arterial diameter at the start of the cardiac cycle. On the basis of the two-dimensional B-mode image, using a 5-MHz probe, an M-line perpendicular to the artery is selected. The radiofrequency signals of four to eight cycles are recorded, digitized, and stored in the memory. Two sample volumes, selected under control of a cursor, are positioned on the anterior and posterior walls of the artery; these volumes track, according to phase, the interfaces selected. Arterial wall displacement is then obtained by autocorrelation processing of the Doppler signals originating from the two sample volumes. High spatial resolution, less than 30 μm for internal diameter and 1 μm for pulsatile change, is achieved. By computing these data, three parameters are obtained: end-diastolic diameter (D_d), absolute stroke change in diameter ($D_s - D_d$), and relative stroke change in diameter ($D_s - D_d)/D_d$. For D_d and $D_s - D_d$ reproducibility is less than 5%.

For the radial artery, an A-mode ultrasonic echo-tracking device (Ansulab SA, Research Laboratories of the SMH Group, Neuchâtel, Switzerland)[33] is used. A 7.5- to 10-MHz focalized transducer is positioned stereotaxically over the artery without contacting the skin. A gel is applied for transmission. The probe is placed perpendicularly to the axis of the artery at its largest cross-sectional dimension, using Doppler mode echocardiography. The transducer is switched to A-mode and the backscattered echoes from both the inner anterior and posterior walls are visualized on an oscilloscope screen. The electric signals of the walls exhibiting a high signal-noise ratio are tagged by an electronic tracer and their movement is tracked. Recording of the tracer's displacement allows derivation of a digitalized signal of diameter change. The inner diameter of the pulsating artery is measured 5000 times per second. High-frequency acquisition of data enables averaging of short series of measurements, which further increases precision of the instrument. The device has been calibrated on artificial targets: resolution is close to 1 μm. The interobserver coefficient of vari-

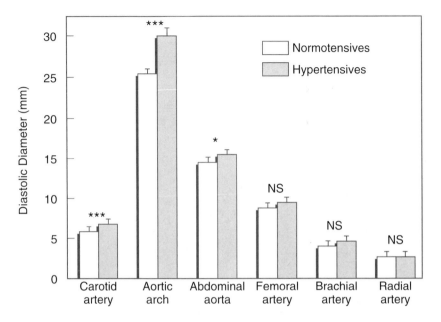

FIGURE 4-1. Diastolic diameter in hypertensive subjects vs. normotensive controls matched for age and sex.[31,36] $p < 0.05$; ***$p < 0.001$.

ation is $2 \pm 2\%$ for D_d, $13 \pm 9\%$ for $D_s - D_d$, and $13 \pm 9\%$ for $(D_s - D_d)/D_d$. Blood pressure may be measured simultaneously at the site of the finger just below the radial artery using a photoplethysmograph (Finapress system. Ohmeda, BOC Group, Inc., Englewood, Colo.). With appropriate modeling pressure-diameter and compliance pressure curves of the radial artery over the cardiac cycle are established.[33]

Values of Arterial Diameter in Subjects with Hypertension

Most age- and sex-adjusted values of diastolic diameter in central and peripheral arteries of both normotensive and hypertensive subjects have been documented under steady-state (i.e., operational steady-state blood pressure) conditions.[31,36] Figure 4-1 shows diastolic arterial diameters in hypertension. The diameters of the carotid artery and aorta are increased. In contrast, no significant change is observed in the brachial, radial, and femoral arteries. The latter do not dilate mechanically in response to the elevated distending pressure and therefore respond actively to the hypertensive process. Since peripheral arteries are primarily muscle tissue, the passive distension caused by the ele-

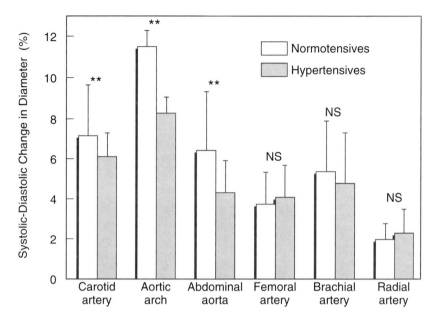

FIGURE 4-2. Arterial diameter changes in systole and diastole $(D_s - D_d/D_d)$ in hypertensive subjects vs. normotensive controls matched by age and sex[31,36]. **$p < 0.01$.

vation in blood pressure should be masked by an associated constriction. The nature of the constrictive response is not known. Endothelial changes may play a role, as suggested by the disturbed response to intra-arterial acetylcholine seen in vivo of the hypertensive forearm.[37,38] It has been noted, however, that in vivo the mechanism of flow dilation or constriction is not impaired at this site.[8] At the same increase in flow velocity, the diameter of the brachial artery increases are similar in both hypertensive and normotensive subjects.

Figure 4-2 shows systolic-diastolic changes in arterial diameter in hypertensive patients and in normotensive controls matched for age and sex.[31,36] In the hypertensive patients, pulsatile changes in the radial, brachial, and femoral arteries are maintained within the range of normal. In contrast, at the sites of the aorta and carotid artery, there is a significant reduction in diameter. In the latter, with the increase in the pulsatile changes of blood pressure (see Fig. 3-2), findings suggest that these arteries develop an active response to the increased mechanical signal. In hypertensive subjects, in fact, a decrease in the pulsatile component of these arteries is observed despite the increase in the pulsatile component of blood pressure.

These findings show that the arteries in hypertensive patients respond actively to blood pressure elevation, as do resistant arteries. These changes in

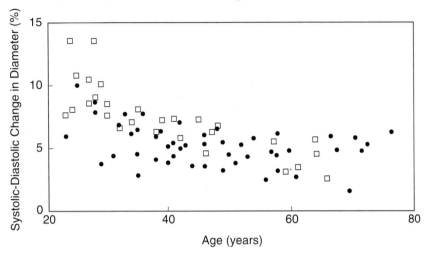

FIGURE 4-3. Age-related pulsatile changes in carotid artery diameter in normotensive *(circles)* and hypertensive *(squares)* populations.[36]

the proximal elastic arteries (aorta, carotid artery) differ from those in the distal muscular (brachial, radial, femoral) components of the arterial system. These findings agree with observations of the effect of age on mechanical properties of arteries.[36] The mechanical properties of the aorta and carotid artery decrease substantially with age (Fig. 4-3). In contrast, this relationship is not seen in the brachial or femoral artery (Fig. 4-4). Thus, in hypertension, the central and peripheral arteries differ greatly in their mechanical properties, especially in response to aging.

INDICES OF ARTERIAL STIFFNESS IN SUBJECTS WITH HYPERTENSION

Our knowledge of arterial stiffness in clinical and experimental hypertension derives from two sources. (i) Studies using complex models of the circulation in humans and laboratory animals have demonstrated that compliance and distensibility of the arterial tree as a whole are reduced in hypertensive subjects.[1,39–41] It is difficult to know, however, whether these changes in compliance and distensibility are related to pressure or to changes that are intrinsic to the arterial wall, or to a combination of these. Comparison of normotensive and hypertensive subjects at the same pressure are difficult to obtain. (ii) Experiments on rings or strips of arterial segments studied in vitro and, in some cases, in vivo[1,5,39,42,43] have demonstrated that increases in carotid and aortic stiffness (particularly

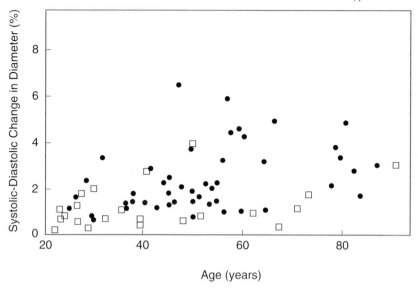

FIGURE 4-4. Age-related pulsatile changes in radial artery diameter in normotensive *(circles)* and hypertensive *(squares)* populations.[3,6]

under full relaxation) are due in part to intrinsic changes of the arterial wall and that these changes are independent of transmural pressure or wall stress changes. The reader is referred to several reviews on the subject.[1–5,39,42,43] Recent investigation of arterial segments in hypertensive humans are presented below.

Indices of Systemic Arterial Stiffness

On the basis of relatively simple arterial models of the circulation, estimates of arterial compliance have been made using analysis of the blood pressure curve. The aortic valves are closed during diastole so the diastolic waveform can be considered as the transient response of the arterial system to the systolic pressure changes.[1,5,40,43–47] In this case, the blood pressure curve commonly assumes a monoexponential form. This aspect of diastolic decay may be evaluated more precisely by determining the areas under the systolic and diastolic portions of the aortic pressure tracing.[40] For the range of frequency of this portion of the tracing, the wavelength is much longer than the length of the arterial tree, and the large artery acts as a pure elastic-compliance chamber (C) branched in series with single resistance (R). Under these conditions, a simple Windkessel model can be used to evaluate compliance. The Windkessel model is analogous to the electrical *RC* model, in which a single capacitance (C) and single resistance (R) are associated in series. Systemic arterial compliance is often approximated to the ratio between the time constant of diastolic decay and calculated vascular resistance.[1,5,40,44] Validations of the model have been suggested in humans,[44] and improvements proposed that would distinguish between distal and proximal compliance.[41] Using the Windkessel model, it has been demonstrated that systemic, or aortic, compliance is consistently reduced in hypertensive subjects.[1,40,41,44] On the basis of the administration of vasoactive drugs, some studies indicate that the reduction in aortic compliance cannot be attributed entirely to the mechanical effect of hypertension but also involve intrinsic changes of the arterial wall.[40,45]

Several criticisms of the methodology of the clinical use of the Windkessel model have been summarized by Yin and Liu.[43] The most important limitation of the Windkessel model is that pressure oscillations are assumed to be synchronous everywhere. The model overlooks the fundamental characteristics of finite wave velocity and definite wave reflection which characterize the living arterial tree.[1] This aspect is particularly important for the study of compliance following administration of vasoactive agents. Such drugs significantly modify wave velocity.[6] In some human arterial segments in which arterial length is short compared with pressure wave length, wave velocity may be considered infinite and the Windkessel model may be used as a first approximation. Levy et al.[46] report that in small rodents, as in spontaneously hypertensive rats, systemic compliance is reduced and correlates strongly with the characteristic impedance calculated from Fourier analysis. The same application may be done in the total vasculature of the forearms of humans; arterial compliance was significantly reduced in hypertensive subjects compared with normal controls matched by age, sex, and pressure.[47]

In addition to the Windkessel model, the rate of propagation of the pressure wave along the arterial system, that is, pulse-wave velocity (PWV), is widely used for estimation of arterial stiffness.[1,2,39] PWV is measured from the foot of pressure waves recorded at two sites on the arterial tree and calculated as L/dt, where L is the distance between the two sites and dt is the time delay. The method has been described extensively.[1,2,39] The reproducibility for aortic pulse-wave velocity is approximately 5%.[12,22] PWV is related to Young's modulus (E) by the Moens–Korteweg equation:

$$PWV^2 = Eh/2pR \qquad [1]$$

where h is arterial thickness, R is internal radius, and p is blood density. PWV usually ranges from 500 to 2000 cm/s. Thus, the higher the PWV, the greater the rigidity of the arterial wall for a given h/R ratio. PWV is significantly increased in hypertensive subjects compared with age-matched normotensive controls (Fig. 4-5) and even compared with young subjects with borderline hypertension.[1,14,48–51] PWV may be determined at different sites along the arterial tree. It increases from the central aorta to the peripheral brachial and femoral arteries. Only aortic PWV increases significantly with age.[12,49] This increase with age is less pronounced or even absent for the upper and lower limbs.

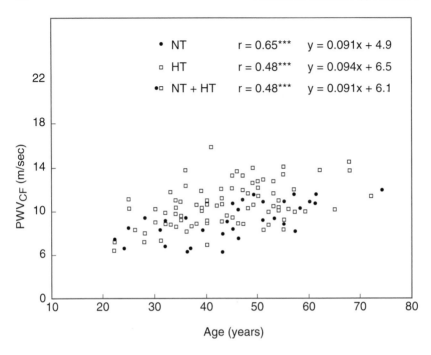

FIGURE 4-5. Carotid-femoral pulse-wave velocity (PWV_{CF}) and age in normotensive and hypertensive subjects (personal data). ***p < 0.001.

Compliance and Distensibility of Arterial Segments

In the forearm, it has been shown, using an airtight box, in hypertensive and normotensive subjects that *PWV* was the same for the same mean arterial pressure. Although this suggests that at the same transmural pressure, arterial distensibility is the same in both groups, the finding may be questioned. According to the Moens–Korteweg equation, an increase in *PWV* may result from an increase in *E* or *h/R*, or a combination of both, and the arterial thickness-internal radius ratio has not been evaluated using an airtight box.

The Moens–Korteweg equation was applied to the measurement of forearm arterial compliance assuming a thin arterial wall.[1,39] In this case, Equation [1] is expressed in terms of compliance (C = $\Delta V/\Delta P$) as:

$$C = \Delta V/\Delta P = V/pPWV^2 \qquad [2]$$

with V artery volume and *h* considered as negligible. When V and $\Delta V/\Delta P$ are expressed by unit length, then Equation [2] becomes:

$$C = 3.14\ R^2/pPWV^2 \qquad [3]$$

Using this method to measure compliance, the internal radius of the brachial artery was measured noninvasively using echo-Doppler techniques and pulse-wave velocity was measured at the same time.[52] This method was used in patients with untreated hypertension who were examined on day 3 of hospitalization; they were found to have the same mean arterial pressure as age- and sex-matched normotensive controls. Forearm arterial compliance was shown under that condition to be significantly reduced in hypertensive subjects. However, the number of subjects was small.

The stiffness of arterial segments may be determined noninvasively in vivo by measuring pulsatile changes in blood pressure and arterial diameter by the applanation tonometric and echo-tracking techniques described in Chapters 3 and 4. It should be noted that the values obtained are limited to the specific site of the arterial segment that is being evaluated and therefore may differ from the in vivo indices of stiffness of all or part of the arterial tree, as derived from the Windkessel model or pulse-wave velocity indices. On the other hand, indices of compliance are evaluated at a given steady-state mean arterial pressure which makes it difficult in most cases to compare normotensive and hypertensive populations at the same transmural pressure. In some cases, the in vivo pressure-diameter relationship, particularly at the site of the radial artery, can be evaluated, which makes a comparison in some cases possible. Again, the findings are difficult to compare with experimental studies in which arterial strips or rings are used in animals. In these studies, normotensive and hypertensive animals were compared at the same transmural pressure, but pulse pressure or pulsatile flow or both were interrupted.

Decreased values of operating distensibility and compliance are found at the site of the central aorta and carotid artery (Figs. 4-6 and 4-7). This agrees with the reduction, described above, in compliance and distensibility determined from cardiovascular models and with in vitro studies using aortic and carotid strips and rings.[1,5,39-43] Comparisons of normotensive and hypertensive subjects for the same transmural pressure showed similar values within the operational blood pressure ranges.[35] In rats, in vitro studies indicate that for the same transmural pressure (below 100–120 mm Hg), carotid artery compliance is reduced in hypertensive animals,[1,5,39-43] but in this preparation flow was stopped.

In the brachial and radial arteries, decreased, and in some cases, normal compliance and distensibility values have been observed (Table 4-1, Figs. 4-6 and 4-7). For the brachial artery, for example, distensibility was reduced but there was no significant change in compliance.[53,54] At this site, however, normotensive and hypertensive subjects could not be compared at the same pressure. Hayoz and colleagues[55] found for the radial artery that compliance was normal or slightly increased in hypertensive vs. normotensive subjects, particularly when measurements were performed for the same blood pressure in both groups.

These variable findings suggest two conclusions: (i) In the presence of elevated blood pressure, mechanical changes in the arteries differ greatly in the central and peripheral compartments. (ii) The results underline the difficulty

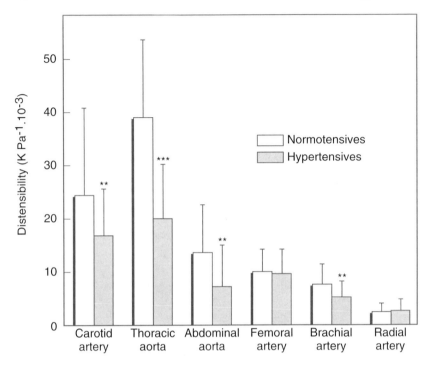

FIGURE 4-6. Indices of operating distensibility in normotensive and hypertensive subjects.[31,36,53] $**p < 0.01$, $*** p < 0.001$.

of obtaining adequate indices of arterial stiffness in humans with hypertension compared with normotensive subjects, at the same transmural pressure. More important, two problems remain to be resolved: (a) it is not only relevant to compare normotensive and hypertensive subjects at the same transmural pressure but also at the same wall stress,[3] and (b) arterial thickness needs to be measured routinely in humans to evaluate more accurate elasticity indices, e.g., the Young modulus (see Chapter 2). Recent studies in hypertensive subjects suggest that the Young modulus might be normal or even decreased.[35]

ARTERIAL THICKENING AND STRUCTURAL CHANGES

The mechanical properties of the arterial wall and, therefore, arterial stiffness, are influenced predominantly by one or more of the structural elements of the artery: endothelium, adventitia, intima, or media.[56] The major contribution of structural components to mechanical properties is assumed to arise from the intima and media, which consist mainly of smooth muscle, elastin, and collagen. The effects of these arterial coats, individually and together, are thought

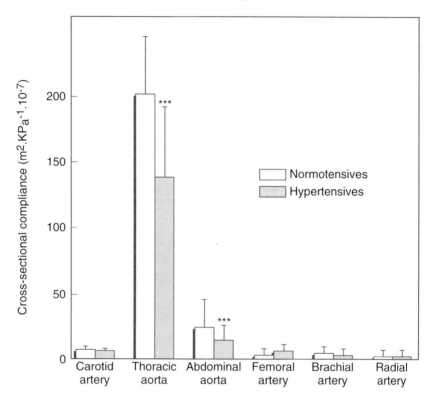

FIGURE 4-7. Indices of operating compliance in normotensive and hypertensive subjects.[31,36,53] ***$p < 0.001$.

to be the primary determinants of the mechanical properties of the vessel wall in its fully relaxed state. This has been clearly demonstrated in various models of experimental hypertension using strips or rings of arteries in vitro and arterial segments in vivo.[1,5,39,42,43] Following total relaxation of arterial smooth muscle, arterial stiffness is increased in hypertensive animals vs. normotensive controls at the same transmural pressure. However, in experimental animals, only the aorta and its major branches have been widely studied.

In order to evaluate the respective roles of smooth muscle, elastin, and collagen on the passive mechanical properties of the arterial wall, Burton[57] showed that Young's modulus for noncontracting smooth muscle was very low, approximately 6×10^4 dynes/cm^2, making it much more extensible than the arterial wall. On the other hand, Young's modulus of isolated elastic tissue was estimated at 3×10^6 dynes/cm^2, and of collagen, approximately 10^9 dynes/cm^2, which indicates that these two components make the principal contribution to the passive mechanical properties of the arterial wall. This assumption was also

TABLE 4-1. *Brachial and radial artery parameters in normotensive and hypertensive subjects*[54]

	NORMOTENSIVES	HYPERTENSIVES
BRACHIAL ARTERY		
Diastolic diameter (D_d) (mm)	4.11 ± 0.7	4.39 ± 0.06
Absolute change in diameter $(D_s–D_d)$ (μm)	193 ± 110	182 ± 104
Relative change in diameter $[D_s–D_d]/D_d]$ (%)	5.03 ± 3.38	4.15 ± 3.00
Distensibility (mm Hg^{-1} · 10^{-3})	1.05 ± 0.82	0.69 ± 0.38*
Cross-sectional compliance (mm^2 · mm Hg^{-1} · 10^{-3})	25.14 ± 16	21.46 ± 12.9
RADIAL ARTERY		
Diastolic diameter (D_d) (mm)	2.87 ± 0.42	2.86 ± 0.55
Absolute change in diameter $(D_s–D_d)$ (μm)	51 ± 23	64 ± 42
Relative change in diameter $[D_s–D_d]/D_d]$ (%)	1.76 ± 0.79	2.33 ± 1.81
Distensibility (mm Hg^{-1} · 10^{-3})	0.33 ± 0.17	0.35 ± 0.31
Cross–sectional compliance (mm^2 · mm Hg^{-1} · 10^{-3})	4.44 ± 2.95	4.38 ± 3.26

±1 standard deviation.
*$p < 0.01$.

illustrated in the experiments of Dobrin et al.[58] who studied isolated human arteries in the presence of elastase and collagenase. With elastase, the pressure-volume relationship of the artery was shifted toward higher values of arterial diameter and volume, which indicates that loss of elastin has a great influence on the cross-sectional area of the artery without modifying its mechanical properties, that is, the slope of the curve. With collagenase, however, there was a considerable change in the slope of the curve, which indicates a decreased wall stiffness without substantial change in diameter and cross-sectional area. Finally, it appears that the passive viscoelastic properties of the arterial wall are chiefly determined by the elastin-collagen ratio. This ratio is greatly influenced by age and hypertension.

Macroscopically, changes in the larger arteries with age support experimental findings (see above). Increases in aortic mass, size of the lumina, and wall thickness have been demonstrated in humans and other animals.[56] These changes are more marked in the subendothelial layer and media, which show an

TABLE 4-2. *Radial artery measurements in hypertensive subjects (personal data)[61]*

	NORMOTENSIVES	HYPERTENSIVES
Age (years)	44.3 ± 11.4	47.9 ± 12.3
Mean arterial pressure (mm Hg)	90.0 ± 14.9	120.9 ± 24.4
Mean diameter (D) (mm)	2.48 ± 0.32	2.53 ± 0.56
Thickness (h) (μm)	204 ± 21	316 ± 53*
$2h/D$ (%)	18 ± 3	26 ± 5*

±1 standard deviation.
*$p < 0.002$.

increase in connective tissue. The most salient changes are the fragmentation and calcification of elastic and the increase in collagen.[56] These findings are predominantly responsible for the age-related increase in pulse-wave velocity (Fig. 4-5). Morphologically, arterial smooth muscle also appears to undergo changes with age, although these changes have not been studied extensively. Age-related changes in the walls of the aorta and carotid artery are accelerated markedly in the presence of hypertension. Age and hypertension both increase aortic smooth muscle and mass collagen content, but the elastin fragmentation and consequent increase in the arterial lumen are more particular to aging.

In humans high-resolution B-mode ultrasonography has been used to estimate changes in carotid artery lesions over time and to quantify normal values.[59,60] Standardized protocols have been established to measure and monitor carotid artery plaque buildup.[60] Reproducibility is considerably improved by performing measurements at various sites: e.g., the distal carotid, the carotid sinus, and the internal carotid artery. About 58.8% of hypertensive patients tested with B-mode ultrasound had carotid intima and media thickness of greater than 1.3 mm, evidence of an abnormality. Carotid artery plaques are found in a high percentage of patients with hypertension, especially in those with elevated systolic pressure. More recent studies have focused on middle-aged subjects with systolic-diastolic hypertension. Echo-Doppler techniques have shown that the thickness of the carotid[59] and radial[61] arteries is significantly increased in hypertensive subjects compared with age- and sex-matched normotensive controls (Table 4-2, Fig. 4-8). The increase in thickness of the radial artery is principally due to an increase in smooth muscle mass. In the carotid and aortic artery walls, increasing amounts of collagen also play a more important role in morphologic and tissue changes and act as a constraining coat once the strain reaches a given level.[1,3,39]

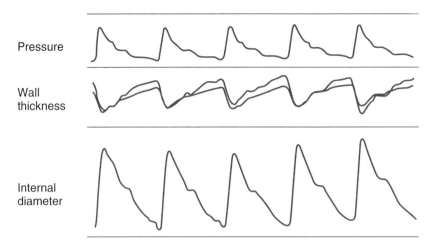

FIGURE 4-8. Echo-Doppler measurements of the internal diameter (systolic-diastolic change) and the wall thickness of the radial artery in a hypertensive subject. Blood pressure was measured at the same time using Finapress.[61]

Morphologic factors figure prominently as to why increased arterial stiffness is found with hypertension in the aorta and major branches. Arterial smooth muscle changes are comparatively of lesser influence, as discussed in Section II of this book. Still, caution should be exercised with regard to this "lesser influence." First, the respective contributions of structural factors and vasomotor tone in maintaining arterial rigidity have not been fully investigated in living animals and humans for the totality of the arterial system. Second, age-related changes in endothelial function and blood pressure may also have an effect on arterial stiffness in hypertension.[62,63] In carotid preparations destruction of endothelium is associated with increased arterial compliance.

AN OVERVIEW

In this chapter important abnormalities in the arterial system of hypertensive persons have been demonstrated. The structural changes are not uniform. The arterial tree may be divided into two compartments—a central compartment and a peripheral compartment. The central compartment comprises the aorta and its major branches; the peripheral compartment comprises the more distal arteries.

Arterial cross-sectional area and volume are increased in the aorta and major branches, with an increase in pulse-wave velocity and a decrease in distensibility. The aorta is predominantly made up of elastic tissue, and therefore these hemodynamic changes in the aorta are highly pressure-dependent. The increase in pressure wave reflections is largely in the central thoracic aorta, which contributes in older subjects to a large increase in pulse pressure and causes a predominant increase in systolic over diastolic pressure in subjects with hypertension. These events are strongly influenced by aging and may lead to development of ventricular hypertrophy,[19,64] with a significant influence on cardiovascular morbidity and mortality as shown by epidemiological studies.[18] In the peripheral arteries in hypertension, there is little change in arterial cross-sectional area and volume and in compliance and distensibility. This may be observed particularly at the site of the radial artery. In subjects with hypertension this difference in diameter between the central aorta and its major branches and the peripheral arteries may contribute to modification of the sites of reflection points with age, making them closer to the heart. Peripheral arteries are predominantly comprised of smooth muscle and thus poorly sensitive to changes in blood pressure, unlike the central arteries, but they change rapidly with modifications in vascular tone, as do resistant arteries.

In hypertension, the heterogeneity of the vascular tree seems to be largely dependent on differences in arterial wall structure.[65] In the central arteries, elastin and collagen predominate over smooth muscle cells, whereas in peripheral arteries smooth muscle and elastin predominate. Thus different ratios are observed between distensible (smooth muscle plus elastin) and nondistensible (collagen) tissue and they will influence the degree of arterial stiffness.

LARGE ARTERIES AND ANTIHYPERTENSIVE DRUG TREATMENT

On the basis of epidemiological studies, [66] it is widely accepted that the level of blood pressure is directly and homogeneously related to the incidence of arterial cerebral, cardiac, and renal complications. In contrast, the effects of drug treatment in therapeutic trials of hypertension clearly showed that the blood pressure reduction was associated with a significant decrease in stroke and congestive heart failure but was substantially less effective on ischemic coronary complications.[66] This observation suggested that drug treatment may modify not only the status of resistant arterioles but also the structure and function of large arteries. For the latter, the beneficial effect of drug treatment is not homogenous. Indeed, the complications of the hypertensive vascular disease are known to be largely related to arterial (atherosclerotic plaques, stenosis, thrombosis, rupture, etc.) rather than to arteriolar damages, and coronary ischemic disease is not considerably improved by drug therapy for hypertension.

In recent years, the response of large arteries to antihypertensive drug treatment has been extensively investigated, with three principal directions. First, it has been recognized that antihypertensive drugs may affect the arterial wall pharmacologically independently of blood pressure changes and that this response varies greatly from one vascular territory to another. Second, antihypertensive therapy and blood pressure reduction affect the structure of the arterial wall. Third, it has been noticed that the aging process modifies the structure and function of large vessels and interferes largely with the effects of long term antihypertensive therapy. Finally, antihypertensive drug treatment is connected with several other vascular risk factors, such as those related to smoking and metabolic abnormalities.

PHARMACOLOGICAL EFFECTS OF ANTIHYPERTENSIVE AGENTS ON THE ARTERIES

SIMPLIFIED BASIC CONCEPTS

Because arterial stiffening in hypertension is heterogeneous and associated with intrinsic modifications of the arterial wall, it is likely that the response by the large arteries to antihypertensive compounds might differ according to the mechanism of action of each particular agent. The comparison of the calcium entry blocker diltiazem with the vasodilator dihydralazine, both administered acutely, gave the first insight indicating that, whereas dihydralazine reduced the brachial artery diameter in hypertensive subjects, diltiazem increased the same arterial calibre for an equivalent blood pressure reduction.[67] Further evidence for a differential action on the brachial artery diameter, despite a similar blood pressure reduction, was obtained by dilatation produced by nitrates[27,28,68] and by angiotensin converting enzyme (ACE) inhibitors;[69,70] yet, blockade of the autonomic nervous system did not markedly modify the cross-sectional area of the vessels.[71] These findings clearly indicated that pressure changes alone cannot explain the modifications seen in arterial diameter following drug treatment of hypertension.

Under drug treatment, numerous factors may simultaneously affect the arterial wall. The most classical factors are the drug-induced relaxing effect on arterial smooth muscle and the passive changes in diameter due to blood pressure changes. The drug-induced counter-regulatory mechanisms, such as those produced by the sympathetic nervous system and the renin-angiotensin system and numerous nonspecific mechanisms related to the myogenic response and flow-dependent dilation also play an important part.[7] For instance, many studies have shown that the elevation of blood flow per se may be responsible for arterial dilation, acting through an endothelium-dependent mechanism that causes the release of vasoactive substances such as NO and endothelin.[7] This mechanism has been observed to operate not only in animals but also in

TABLE 5-1. *Studies on changes in arterial compliance following treatment with antihypertensive agents*[a]

TREATMENT STUDIES	CLINICAL STUDIES	EXPERIMENTAL STUDIES	COMPLIANCE INCREASE
ACE inhibitors	69,70,72,89	42,63	Major
Calcium entry blockers	73,74,92	75	
Nitrates and derivatives	27,28,76	71,27	
α-blockade	77	78,79	Intermediate
Selective B-blockade	80,81	84	
B-blockade with ancillary properties	71,82,83,	84	
Diuretics, salt restriction	50,85,86	87,88	Minor
Nonselective B-blockade	71,89	84	
Dihydralazine and derivatives	90		
Central antihypertensive agents	91		

[a]The number indicates the corresponding reference; in clinical studies, only randomized trials are indicated here.
ACE, angiotensin converting enzyme.

the forearms of normotensive and hypertensive subjects.[8] Reactive hyperemia following wrist occlusion is associated with a consistent increase in brachial artery diameter as a consequence of the distal arteriolar dilation and the resulting increase in flow velocity. For instance, high flow dilation at the site of the brachial artery may partly contribute to the increase in arterial diameter that has been observed following ACE inhibition.[72]

As resulting from drug-induced changes of the arterial wall, not only the diameter of the vessel is modified but also the viscoelastic properties of the arterial wall. Both clinical and animal studies have been performed on this subject (Table 5-1). Most of them have been done on the human brachial artery and on the rat carotid artery, both in acute and in long-term situations[27,28,42,50,69–92] and reviewed in reference 71. In this review, only clinical data will be analyzed in detail.

CONVERTING ENZYME INHIBITORS

Studies were performed with healthy volunteers and hypertensive subjects.[69–72,89] When healthy volunteers were maintained on a double-blind design versus place-

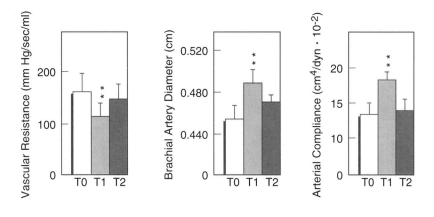

T0 = before treatment
T1 = following one month of perindopril
T2 = following one month of placebo

T1 was significantly (** p<0.01) different from T0 and T2.

FIGURE 5-1. Effects of long-term treatment by perindopril on brachial artery diameter and compliance and forearm vascular resistance in comparison with placebo (mean ± SEM). (Modified from Asmar RG et al.[70])

bo, increasing doses of the converting enzyme inhibitor perindopril caused a preferential vasodilating effect on arterioles at the lower dose; the diameter enhancement of the brachial artery required doses that were two- to three-fold higher. In patients with sustained essential hypertension, acute long-term oral administration of captopril, enalapril, and perindopril also caused a significant diameter enhancement (Fig. 5-1). As such findings were observed in the presence of a significant reduction in blood pressure, it appeared that the mechanical effects of blood pressure were offset by the arterial dilating effect of converting enzyme inhibition. Thus, in humans, converting enzyme inhibitors were able to modify the arterial wall independently of blood pressure.

In addition to the increased arterial diameter, studies in patients with essential hypertension showed a significant increase in arterial compliance, as observed in the systemic and in the brachial circulations following converting enzyme inhibition by captopril, enalapril, and perindopril.[69–72,89] It was suggested that, in addition to blood pressure reduction, the effect of converting enzyme inhibition on arterial smooth muscle caused a relaxation of the arterial wall, with a resulting increase in compliance, as observed in animal hypertension.[42,63] This suggestion was supported by the finding that the increase in arterial compliance following perindopril in hypertensive humans was not associated with a change in the tangential tension of the arterial wall, thus minimizing the role of mechanical and geometrical factors in the development of compliance enhancement. This interpretation is further reinforced by a double-blind randomized study comparing the effect on blood pressure reduction and on arterial compliance of two drug regimens, perindopril and hydrochlorothiazide-amiloride. Although antihypertensive efficacy was equal in both groups, perindopril significantly improved carotid and femoral compliance and distensibility, whereas the diuretic had no effect[92a] (see Fig. 5-2).

CALCIUM-ENTRY BLOCKERS

In a double-blind study involving healthy volunteers (see review in references 71 and 74) increasing doses of the calcium-entry blocker nicardipine increased the brachial and common carotid artery diameter in a dose-dependent manner. No significant modification was observed with a placebo. Systemic blood pressure did not change, suggesting that the calcium-entry blocker acted on the arterial wall independently of pressure-induced mechanical changes. Interestingly, the calcium-entry blocker verapamil did not increase arterial diameter in healthy volunteers, although blood pressure was affected slightly and significantly decreased.

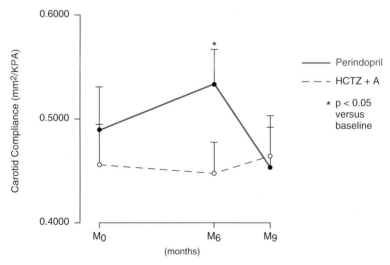

FIGURE 5-2. Carotid compliance of hypertensive patients treated in a double-blind randomized fashion 6 months with perindopril (*n* = 17) or hydrochlorothiazide + amiloride HCTZ + A (*n* = 19) followed by a 3-month placebo run-out period. The diastolic blood pressure decrease was significant and similar in both treatment groups. Compliance was significantly increased with perindopril after 6 months of treatment whereas it was not modified with the HCTZ + A treatment.[92a]

In patients with sustained essential hypertension,[74] acute single oral administration of diltiazem and of various dihydropiridine derivatives—for example, nifedipine, nicardipine and nitrendipine—caused a significant increase in arterial diameter of the brachial but not of the carotid artery. With oral nitrendipine, the increase in brachial diameter was shown to be maintained from several weeks. As such findings were again obtained in the presence of a significant reduction in blood pressure, it was clear that the dilating arterial effects of calcium inhibition were not secondary to the blood pressure reduction itself.

In addition to changes in arterial diameter, arterial compliance may also be modified by calcium blockade.[74,92] Short-term and long-term administration of dihydropiridine derivatives to patients with essential hypertension caused a significant increase in arterial compliance and distensibility, both in the systemic and in the brachial circulations.

The mechanism for the increase in arterial compliance was difficult to analyze and might result from several possibilities.[74] First, the blood pressure reduction itself could favor the compliance enhancement through a lower stretch on the arterial wall. Second, because the circumferential elasticity of a blood vessel is related to its radius rather than to the pressure itself, the increase in arterial diameter could play a role *per se*, thus contributing to reduce compliance. Finally, the drug effect on arterial smooth muscle could favor the relaxation of the arterial wall.[75] It is therefore important to evaluate the respective roles of the mechanical (blood pressure) and geometrical (arterial diameter) factors associated to the changes in arterial compliance produced by calcium inhibitors.

To respond to this question, acute blood pressure reduction due to arteriolar vasodilatation was produced in hypertensives using three different pharmacological agents, cadralazine (a dihydralazine-like compound),[90] nicorandil (a nicotinamide derivative), and nitrendipine (a calcium-entry blocker).[74] For an equipotent reduction in blood pressure, cadralazine significantly reduced brachial artery diameter, whereas nicorandil and nitrendipine increased it. Nitrendipine and nicorandil significantly increased arterial compliance, which was not modified by cadralazine. Thus, in essential hypertension, drug-induced changes in the arterial wall cannot be entirely due to pressure changes and may be mediated by predominant geometrical modifications (cadralazine or nicorandil) or by the predominant relaxing effect of the drug on arterial smooth muscle tone (nitrendipine) or by a combination of both factors.

NITRATES AND DERIVATIVES

Animal studies have shown that nitrates exert a preferential action in the larger arteries as opposed to the smaller coronary arteries.[71] Similar observations are also found in humans.[27,28,76] Angiographic investigations in coronary heart failure have shown that nitrates preferentially dilate large coronary arteries, acting both on stenotic and nonstenotic segments. In hypertensive subjects, noninvasive studies using pulsed Doppler and echographic devices indicated that dilation of the brachial arteries, the common carotid arteries, and the aortic arch occur almost constantly following intravenous nitroglycerine or oral isosorbide dinitrate. The resulting dilation approximates 20% in the brachial artery, 9% in the common carotid artery, and only 4% in the aortic arch. The vasodilating effect occurs even when a significant decrease in systolic, diastolic, and mean arterial pressure is observed, suggesting a specific drug-induced mechanism acting on the hypertensive arterial wall. At the site of the brachial and the carotid arteries, large artery dilation is observed without any significant change in vascular resistance and in cross-sectional blood flow velocity, indicating that the mechanism of high flow dilation was not operating after nitrate administration.

The drug-induced effect on the vessel diameter is not a sufficient explanation for the predominant or selective decrease in systolic blood pressure usually produced by nitrates. An increase in arterial compliance and distensibility and/or a change in the timing of wave reflections should also be demonstrated. For this purpose, the induced blood pressure changes produced by nitroglycerine were controlled as a variable by performing measurements with the subject's forearm in a plastic cylinder at a variety of cylinder pressures.[76] Using this method, nitroglycerine infusion was shown to increase forearm arterial distensibility at every pressure, thus demonstrating that nitrates improved arterial stiffness independently of pressure changes. Finally, accepting that arterial compliance is the product of arterial volume by distensibility, it is clear that the nitrate-induced changes in arterial compliance depend principally on the relative amplitude of the changes in vessel geometry and distensibility in each particular situation. As for a given arterial smooth muscle activity, a vessel becomes stiffer when it is distended; arterial compliance is expected to be enhanced when there is a small increase in arterial diameter and a large decrease in pulse-wave velocity and poorly modified in the inverse situation.

ALPHA- AND BETA-ADRENERGIC BLOCKING AGENTS

The action of beta-adrenoreceptors on the large arteries[80–84,89] depends on the class of the beta-blocker and the artery studied. The forearm arterial effects of propranolol and enalapril were compared by dual-crystal pulsed Doppler in patients with essential hypertension.[89] Although the antihypertensive action of the two drugs was similar, only enalapril increased the brachial artery diameter and compliance. Propranolol did not induce any arterial change. Similar results have been reported after acute intravenous administration of propranolol: in young patients with isolated systolic hypertension, propranolol did not change the arterial compliance, despite a significant antihypertensive action related to a decrease in ventricular ejection; in older patients with isolated systolic hypertension, propranolol did not change the blood pressure but induced a significant decrease in compliance. In another study, propranolol and pindolol were compared.[71,84] After a 3-month period the two drugs caused a similar decrease in blood pressure, but different effects on forearm arterial hemodynamics were observed. While propranolol did not induce any change, pindolol produced an increase in brachial artery diameter and compliance. As pindolol also induced a decrease in vascular resistance, it was difficult to conclude whether the vasodilation of the brachial artery was the consequence of the alteration of the microvasculature or of the partial agonist activity of pindolol.[71,84]

Results concerning the use of beta-one cardioselective drugs are contradictory and vary according to the artery studied. Bisoprolol was associated with a decrease in arterial pulse-wave velocity and an increase in brachial artery compliance (Fig. 5-3),[80] and nebivolol was associated with an increase in carotid artery distensibility and compliance.[92] However, it has been reported that metoprolol and celiprolol did not influence the diameter and/or the compliance of the brachial artery.[81,82]

Brachial artery hemodynamics were studied in essential hypertensive patients before and after intravenous infusion of urapidil, a drug with hybrid action involving postsynaptic alpha blockade.[77] Urapidil produced a significant drop in blood pressure, with a significant decrease in arteriolar resistance. Brachial artery blood flow increased, whereas brachial artery diameter and compliance did not change significantly. Distensibility increased slightly. Animal studies have shown that alpha blockade acts on the arterial wall independently of blood pressure changes.[78,79]

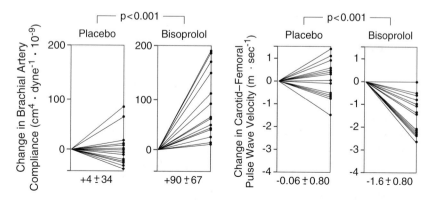

FIGURE 5-3. Changes in brachial artery compliance and carotid femoral wave velocity after bisoprolol and placebo.[80]

Forearm arterial hemodynamics were studied before and after acute administration of the alpha-beta blocking agent, labetalol, in middle-aged patients with essential hypertension.[83] Labetalol caused a significant and rapid drop in blood pressure with a decrease in forearm vascular resistance and an increase in forearm blood flow. Brachial artery diameter did not change, while the brachial artery compliance increased. A similar results was observed following a long-term treatment with the alpha-beta blocking drug medroxalol. Such studies suggest that a combination of alpha and beta blockade produces a higher effect on the arterial wall than separated alpha or beta blockade. The predominant role of alpha receptors for compliance changes may be inferred from the effect of their stimulation on brachial artery diameter in hypertensive subjects. Both norepinephrine infusion and lower body vegative pressure produce a significant decrease in brachial artery diameter.[6, 71]

SODIUM- AND DIURETIC-INDUCED CHANGES IN ARTERIAL DIAMETER AND STIFFNESS

In recent years, three longitudinal studies[85] have focused on sodium-induced changes in arterial diameter and stiffness in different types of hypertensive conditions: mild to moderate essential hypertension in the young to middle aged, systolic hypertension in the elderly and dialyzed patients with end-stage renal disease.

The hemodynamic effect of a moderately low-salt diet was investigated in a two-month randomly allocated, double-blind crossover study in 20 hypertensive ambulatory patients. Blood pressure was significantly lower during the low, compared to the normal-sodium period, but the blood pressure changes were relatively small. However, the brachial artery diameter was significantly larger during the low-sodium period, whereas the carotid artery diameter was unchanged. The changes in brachial artery diameter were not related to blood pressure changes but were positively related to the age of the patients.

Further support for the arterial effect of sodium was obtained from the intravenous administration of isotonic saline (2 liters in 120 min) to elderly subjects with systolic hypertension and arteriosclerosis obliterans of the lower limbs. In these patients, the isotonic saline caused a significant decrease in forearm arterial compliance in parallel with an increase in systolic blood pressure, with no change in diastolic blood pressure, suggesting again that the reduction in arterial compliance following the isotonic saline was due to sodium-induced mechanisms acting on the arterial wall independently of the changes in blood pressure. Similar observations have been made in patients with severe hypertension and end-stage renal disease undergoing hemodialysis. In such subjects, without antihypertensive drug treatment, pulse-wave velocity was increased and was strongly associated with positive sodium balance, as assessed from the interdialytic weight gain. This finding was independent of age and blood pressure levels. During long-term treatment with the calcium blocker nitrendipine, blood pressure decreased rapidly. Pulse wave velocity also decreased significantly but the decrease occurred later and therefore was poorly correlated with the blood pressure reduction. Again, the changes in pulse-wave velocity were strongly associated with the interdialytic weight changes, indicating strong interactions between sodium balance and arterial stiffness in this particular population.

The effect of diuretics on arterial stiffness in hypertension are documented in a small number of studies, one with hydrochlorothiazide and the other with indapamide.[50,71,85,86] The antihypertensive and arterial effects of the diuretic compound hydrochlorothiazide were compared to those of the calcium-entry blocker felodipine in patients with essential hypertension in a double-blind crossover study. Whereas felodipine decreased blood pressure more substantially than hydrochlorothiazide and improved arterial distensibility in the aorta and the upper and lower limbs, the diuretic compound had absolutely no arterial effect despite a significant blood pressure reduction (Table 5-2). In another study using indapamide, systemic arterial compliance increased following drug treatment in a population of subjects with essential hypertension.

TABLE 5-2. *Arterial changes following treatment with hydrochloro-thiazide versus felodipine in a crossover study in subjects with essential hypertension*[86]

	BASELINE	FELODIPINE	HYDRO-CHLOROTHIAZIDE
Systolic blood pressure (mm Hg)	162 ± 12	140 ± 17	150 ± 13**
Diastolic blood pressure (mm Hg)	96 ± 9	85 ± 9	89 ± 9*
Carotid-femoral pulse wave velocity (m/s)	10.9 ± 2.0	9.2 ± 1.8	10.1 ± 2***
Femoro-tibial pulse wave velocity (m/s)	12.8 ± 1.7	11.1 ± 1.9	12.2 ± 1.7***
Carotid-radial pulse wave velocity (m/s)	11.7 ± 1.9	10.0 ± 2	11.8 ± 1.8***
Brachial artery diameter (cm)	0.437 ± 0.06	0.449 ± 0.06	0.431 ± 0.05*
Brachial vascular resistance (dyn/s · cm^{-4})	104 ± 40	72 ± 30	92 ± 46*
Brachial artery compliance (dyn/cm^4 · 10^{-7})	1.13 ± 0.48	1.71 ± 0.83	1.19 ± 0.57***

*$p < 0.05$, **$p < 0.01$, *** $p < 0.001$ (hydrochlorothiazide versus felodipine).

However, the indapamide effect on systemic compliance was not observed in other arteries, such as the brachial artery.

Finally, sodium undoubtedly affects the arterial wall, independently of blood pressure changes. However, the arterial modifications produced by diuretic agents are relatively small in hypertensive humans, and this aspect remains difficult to explain because larger effects are observed in animals.[87,88] Potassium changes are an unlikely explanation, because indapamide and canrenone, which have opposing effects on serum potassium, produce the same arterial changes. Because indapamide had more substantial arterial effects than hydrochlorothiazide, differences in the biochemical structure and/or the drug dose may be involved. However, the best explanation results from two observations. First, the antihypertensive effect of diuretic is modest, with very small possibilities of producing a passive increase in arterial compliance. Second, diuretics activate counter-regulatory mechanisms (including those of the renin-angiotensin system and of the autonomic nervous system), which favor increased arterial rigidity.

DRUG-INDUCED CHANGE IN WAVE REFLECTIONS

Many drugs used in the treatment of cardiovascular diseases exert their action by changing the intensity or timing of wave reflections brought about by alterations in vascular properties. In clinical studies of vasoactive drugs, the radial or brachial arterial pressure are assumed to reflect pressure changes in the overall arterial tree. As we mentioned, this assumption can be accepted for the mean blood pressure, which remains almost constant along the conduit arteries, but not for systolic and pulse pressures, which are amplified toward the periphery by wave reflections. The effect of wave reflection on the augmentation of late systolic pressure is seen in the carotid pressure wave, the ascending aortic pressure wave, and the left ventricular pressure wave in mature humans.[1,71] In contrast, the systolic fluctuation due to wave reflection occurs later in peripheral arteries than it does in central arteries, contributing little or nothing to the systolic peak and pulse pressure amplitude.[1,71] This is an important point, because therapeutic efficiency of drugs is interpreted from pressure recordings in brachial artery, which do not necessarily reflect pressure changes in central arteries. Indeed, drugs that decrease or delay wave reflections would decrease aortic pressure (largely influenced by reflected waves) more than brachial or peripheral systolic and pulse pressure (less or not influenced by wave reflections). Recent studies with antihypertensive drug treatment have indeed shown that changes in systolic and pulse pressure in aorta and central arteries could be induced by various drug regimens independently of changes in pressure in peripheral arteries.[1,71]

Studies of pulsatile arterial hemodynamics indicate that antihypertensive agents do not only affect mean blood pressure but may also induce important in the pulsatile component of blood pressure dissociated from changes in mean pressure. The antihypertensive drugs (and vasodilators in general) can change the intensity and/or the timing of wave reflection by several mechanisms.[1,71] The decrease in the intensity of wave reflection could be due to decreased peripheral resistance and decreased reflection coefficient,[1-3] or to an increase in the cross-sectional area ratio at arterial branching by dilation of smaller conduit arteries proximal to arterioles. An alteration in the timing of wave reflection could be achieved by delaying the return of reflected waves and/or to a lesser degree by shortening the ventricular ejection. The delay in the return of reflected wave results from a decrease in arterial pulse wave velocity, whether related to a decrease in blood pressure or to eventual alterations of the intrinsic viscoelastic properties of arterial walls.

With antihypertensive therapy in man, changes in arterial pressure wave contour and impedance are usually due to a combination of effects on the intensity and timing of wave reflections. Antihypertensive agents with vasodilator properties (nitroprusside, ACE inhibitors, calcium channel blockers) reduce intensity of wave reflection by arteriolar vasodilation (decreased peripheral resistances) and by delay in the return of reflected waves (decreased pulse wave velocity).[1,71] As the reflected wave in mature adult humans constitutes the late systolic peak in central but not in peripheral arteries, the pressure recorded in brachial artery underestimates the pressure changes in the aorta and left ventricle. By contrast with vasodilating drugs, propranolol increases vascular resistance and wave reflections.[45] Atenolol, a beta-blocking agent without vasodilator properties, increases peripheral resistances and intensity of wave reflections.[1,71] It decreases the aortic pulse wave velocity and delays the return of reflected wave.[1,71] This potentially beneficial effect is offset by the brachycardia and parallel increase in the duration of left ventricular ejection. On the other hand, the beta-blocking agent dilevalol consistently reduces the intensity of wave reflections with a resultant greater fall in central aortic systolic pressure compared to atenolol.[71]

As we showed in Chapter 3, the effect of nitrates, which are widely used in cardiovascular medicine, appears to be strikingly different from the previously mentioned drugs. Indeed, the previously mentioned vasodilator and antihypertensive agents act by combined effect on the intensity and timing of wave reflection, decreasing blood pressure and pulse wave velocity and reducing the peripheral resistances. Nitroglycerin decreases the ascending aortic and left ventricular pressure. This effect is not caused by arteriolar dilatation and fall in peripheral resistances, and it may occur without substantial change in aortic distensibility and/or pulse wave velocity.[1,71] The major effect of nitrates is to decrease the intensity of reflected wave but without decreasing terminal (arteriolar) reflection coefficient. Nitrates do that by increasing the caliber and distensibility of small conduit arteries proximal to the arterioles, thereby increasing the cross-sectional area ratio at these arterial branching sites, thus decreasing the distance between the heart and reflection sites and therefore the amplitude of reflected waves at this level. As with other drugs that reduce wave reflections, the effect of nitrates on systolic pressure is more pronounced in the ascending aorta and in central arteries than in peripheral arteries.

A SIMPLE OVERVIEW OF THE ARTERIAL CHANGES PRODUCED BY ANTIHYPERTENSIVE AGENTS

Studies of pharmacological agents clearly indicate that for the same blood pressure reduction, arterial stiffness may be modified to a greater or lesser extent depending on the antihypertensive compound (Table 5-1). A marked increase in compliance is obtained with ACE inhibitors, such as perindopril, calcium entry blockers, and nitrates. Intermediate changes are obtained with blockade of the autonomic nervous system, particularly following alpha- and beta-one blockade. Minor changes are observed with diuretic compounds, noncardioselective beta blocking agents such as propranolol, and dihydralazine (or derivatives). Thus, vasodilating compounds may have various effects on large and small vessels, leading to different hemodynamic patterns on forearm vessels following antihypertensive therapy: decreased vascular resistance and increased arterial stiffness (as with dihydralazine and derivatives and propranolol) or decreased vascular resistance and reduced arterial stiffness (as with nitrates, ACE inhibitors, and calcium entry blockers).

Nevertheless, an important aspect of the drug effect on the arterial system is the heterogeneity of the response according to the territories involved. For instance, nitrates increase compliance at the site of the carotid artery and distensibility at the site of the brachial artery, whereas both changes are observed at the site of the femoral artery.[28] Again, the structure and the function of each particular artery influence greatly the drug-induced changes in the mechanical properties of the arteries.

6

ARTERIES AND LONG-TERM ANTIHYPERTENSIVE THERAPY

STRUCTURAL CHANGES OF THE ARTERIES FOLLOWING ANTIHYPERTENSIVE DRUG TREATMENT

In considering the arterial response to antihypertensive therapy, it is important to notice that, with long-term treatment, structural changes of the arterial wall (either due to the blood pressure reduction or to the drug effect or to a combination of both factors) may be associated with blood pressure changes. This important aspect has been particularly studied following converting enzyme inhibition in various models of Goldblatt rats and spontaneously hypertensive rats.[6,42,63] Together with the reduction of cardiac hypertrophy, a reduction of aortic medial thickness is observed, principally due to a decrease in the amount of arterial smooth muscle. These structural changes are associated with an increase in systemic and carotid arterial compliance.

In hypertensive humans, such changes are more difficult to assess, because measurements of the thickness of the arterial wall are not easy to obtain. Direct structural assessment of resistant arteries has only recently been made possible using the Mulvany-Halpern myograph.[93,93a] It could be shown on biopsies of gluteal arterioles that a 9-month perindopril treatment normalized media-to-lumen ratio.[93] Interestingly, this effect was independent of blood pressure reduction as infered from another double-blind randomized study comparing perindopril and atenolol (see Fig. 6-1). Although blood pressure was decreased to the same extent in both groups, perindopril significantly reduced media-to-lumen ratio whereas atenolol had no effect on the media-to-lumen

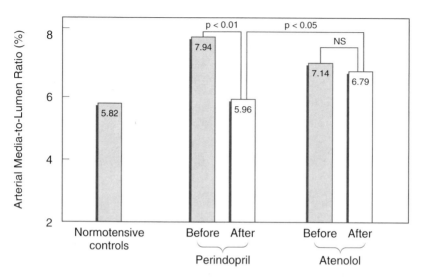

FIGURE 6-1. Changes in media-to-lumen ratio of small resistance vessels of hypertensive patients after a one-year treatment. Although the same blood pressure reduction was achieved with perindopril ($n=13$) and atenolol ($n=12$), only the former drug corrected media-to-lumen ratio as well.[93a]

ratio.[93a] On the other hand, it has been noticed that, following converting enzyme inhibition in hypertensive subjects, there is no strict parallelism between the blood pressure reduction, the reversion of cardiac hypertrophy, and the large artery compliance changes.[70,72] Whereas the blood pressure reduction is rapid, the regression of cardiovascular structural changes is of longer duration, with different time constants for the heart and arterial vessels. For the heart, two months may be sufficient to reduce cardiac hypertrophy; the change is even maintained when treatment is stopped for one month. This effect on cardiac hypertrophy with perindopril [70,72] was not observed with a calcium entry blocker.[93b] For the arterial vessels, the reversion probably needs a much longer duration. Indeed, the regression of collagen fibers is difficult to obtain, due to the long turnover of this material.

Recently, radial artery thickness was measured in hypertensive subjects submitted to long term antihypertensive therapy.[94] Both cross-sectional and longitudinal studies were performed. In a cross-sectional study, the radial thickness was shown to be increased in untreated hypertensive subjects and to remain within the normal range in well-controlled hypertensive subjects submitted to various forms of antihypertensive therapy. In a longitudinal study comparing a diuretic agent and a converting enzyme inhibitor in a double-blind trial, radial artery thickness was shown to be reduced by treatment in proportion to the decrease in blood pressure. Nevertheless, for the interpretation of the results, it should be recognized that the radial artery is composed principally of arterial smooth muscle and that the comparison with another artery involving more important amounts of collagen may give different information.

LONG-TERM DRUG TREATMENT OF HYPERTENSION IN RELATION TO THE AGING PROCESS

Because drug treatment of hypertension is of long duration, the effectiveness of therapy should be analyzed in parallel with the study of the aging process. In this context, it is well accepted that blood pressure increases with age.[1] However, systolic blood pressure increases much more with age than does diastolic blood pressure, particularly in females. Diastolic blood pressure even tends to fall in those over 70 years of age. Subsequently, mean arterial pressure increases slightly with age whereas pulse pressure increases more markedly, particularly after 70 years of age. These age-related changes in blood pressure indicate that arterial stiffness and wave reflections increase much more with age than does vascular resistance.[1] Such hemodynamic aspects of the normal aging process may explain several features of the long-term treatment of hypertension, particularly in groups of subjects in which diastolic blood pressure is controlled by drug therapy, whereas systolic blood pressure remains uncontrolled.

In order to evaluate the role of the aging process following antihypertensive drug treatment, an example will be given in subjects with hypertension. The mechanical properties of the common carotid artery (CCA) were investigated in a study comparing 46 normotensive subjects and 81 age-matched hypertensive patients.[95] The latter group included 25 patients well controlled (systolic blood pressure < 160 mmHg; diastolic blood pressure < 90 mmHg) by antihypertensive drug treatment for at least 3 months and 56 untreated hypertensives. Antihypertensive therapy was based on a stepped-care approach involving diuretics, beta-blocking agents, and vasodilators. The three groups did not differ with respect to age, total or high-density lipoprotein plasma cholesterol and plasma glucose, and smoking.

Table 6-1 shows that arterial diameter and the Peterson elastic modulus (i.e., the inverse of distensibility; see page 16) were increased in subjects with untreated hypertension. In well-controlled hypertensives, the Peterson modulus was slightly increased but the diastolic diameter was within the normal range. In each group, there were significant expected relationships between age and CCA dimensional and functional data, including end-diastolic diameter, absolute and relative stroke changes in diameter and the Peterson elastic modulus, indicating a widening of the CCA with advancing age and a decrease in its buffering function. When compared with untreated hypertensives, well-controlled hypertensives had significantly lower values of blood pressure and the Peterson modulus. However, the most important findings appeared

TABLE 6-1. *Blood pressure and common carotid artery dimensional data*[95]

	I NORMOTENSIVE SUBJECTS (N = 46)	II WELL CONTROLLED HYPERTENSIVE PATIENTS (N = 25)	III UNTREATED HYPERTENSIVE PATIENTS (N = 58)
Systolic blood pressure (mm Hg)	129.9 ± 12.6 ***	131.8 ± 11.4***	155.9 ± 13.1
Diastolic blood pressure (mm Hg)	80.9 ± 7.8***	76.5 ± 9.6 **	94.8 ± 8.6
Mean arterial pressure (mm Hg)	96.9 ± 8.4***	94.8 ± 8.6***	115.0 ± 8.7
Pulse pressure (mm Hg)	48.9 ± 9.7***	55.2 ± 11.8**	61.4 ± 11.9
Heart rate (beats/min)	68.7 ± 11.2	68.2 ± 18.9	67.4 ± 9.4
Common carotid artery			
D_d (mm)	6.9 ± 0.9**	7.2 ± 0.9	7.4 ± 0.9
$D_s - D_d$ (mm)	0.42 ± 0.00	0.39 ± 0.2	0.40 ± 0.13
$[(D_s - D_d)/D_d]$ (%)	6.1 ± 1.6	5.5 ± 1.9	5.5 ± 1.9
E_p (dyn/cm$^2 \cdot 10^6$)	1.14 ± 0.42***	1.46 ± 0.53	1.72 ± 0.86

Values are expressed as means ± standard deviation.
$*p < 0.05$, $**p < 0.01$, $***p < 0.001$, versus Group III.
D_d, end-diastolic diameter; $D_s - D_d$, stroke change in diameter during systole; $(D_s - D_d/D_d$, relative stroke change in diameter; E_p, pressure-strain elastic modulus (Peterson modulus).

when the Peterson elastic modulus was related to age (Fig. 6-2). At any given value of age, the modulus was higher in hypertensive than in normotensive subjects. This finding was observed even in well-controlled hypertensives, indicating that, with efficient antihypertensive therapy, the carotid arterial wall remained stiffer than it did in controls and that the increase in arterial stiffness with age was substantially steeper than in normotensive subjects.

For understanding these findings, it is thus important to recall that, following long-term antihypertensive therapy, two different processes are involved: the hypertensive process and the aging process. As we mentioned, the aging process tends per se to increase systolic blood pressure and to decrease diastolic blood pressure at any given value of mean arterial pressure, due to the progressive increase in arterial stiffening with age. However, independently of age, antihypertensive drug treatment tends to decrease diastolic blood pressure through arteriolodilatation and decrease mean arterial pressure. When the two processes are combined, both of them contribute to a decrease in diastolic blood pressure, whereas only the aging process tends to maintain or even increase systolic

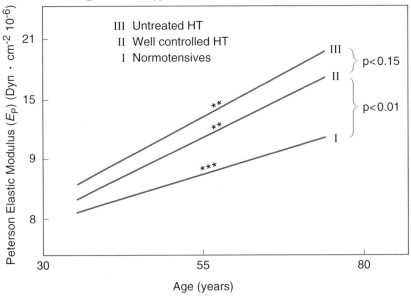

FIGURE 6-2. Relationship between the Peterson elastic modulus *(E_P)* and age in normotensive subjects (Group I), in untreated hypertensive subjects (Group II), and in well-controlled hypertensive subjects following drug therapy (Group III).[95]

blood pressure and hence pulse pressure. Possibly for that reason, a substantial number of subjects with treated hypertension have a controlled diastolic blood pressure but an elevated systolic blood presure. Finally, it appears clear that diastolic blood pressure should not be the exclusive criterion used to evaluate the beneficial effect of antihypertensive therapy. Not only diastolic blood pressure but also systolic blood pressure should be reduced and fully controlled with long-term treatment.

INFLUENCE OF TOBACCO CONSUMPTION AND METABOLIC ABNORMALITIES ON ARTERIAL STIFFNESS

Cardiovascular risk is not only mediated by high blood pressure but also by smoking and by several metabolic abnormalities involving plasma insulin, glucose, lipids, and calcium. Till this chapter, we have not discussed the fact that smoking and metabolic factors should be taken into account in the hemodynamic changes of the hypertensive large arteries. However, these factors may act on the arterial wall with several consequences. First,excess tobacco consumption and metabolic abnormalities per se are frequently associated with increased arterial stiffness. Second, important interactions may be observed between these metabolic disturbances and antihypertensive drug therapy, a finding that is known to be influenced by the pharmacological characteristics of the drug used. Finally, hypertension and atherosclerosis are frequently associated and may both contribute independently to arterial stiffening.

RELATIONSHIP OF SMOKING AND METABOLIC DISORDERS TO ARTERIAL STIFFNESS

This review includes a discussion of the following factors: smoking, cholesterol excess, increased plasma glucose and insulin, and calcifications and abnormalities of the calcium metabolism.

Smoking
Whereas smoking is known to alter the arterial wall and particularly the endothelial function, few studies have been done on the influence of increased tobacco consumption on arterial stiffness. Acute smoking in healthy volunteers

not only increases blood pressure and heart rate but also pulse-wave velocity.[96] On the other hand, in epidemiologic studies, it has been generally admitted that occasional blood pressure measurements are somewhat lower in smokers than in nonsmokers. But, in these studies it is important to consider that subjects did not smoke at the time of the blood pressure measurements. However, when ambulatory rather than occasional blood pressure measurements are performed, it appears that a different picture may be observed.[97] With ambulatory blood pressure measurements, blood pressure is higher in smokers than in nonsmokers, and this increase is found principally in systolic pressure and pulse pressure. Interestingly, this hemodynamic pattern is observed only during day time and disappears during the night (i.e., in the absence of smoking). Thus, smoking is one of the factors that may contribute to increased pulse-wave velocity and pulse pressure, at least acutely.

Cholesterol excess

Based on experimental and clinical studies, it has been reported that cholesterol excess substantially alters the endothelial function, leading to a decreased relaxation of the arterial vessels.[98] The defect has been described mainly in atherosclerotic patients, but it has also been described in asymptomatic subjects with hypercholesterolemia.[99] Whether this abnormality is associated with an increased stiffness of the arterial wall in humans remains to be demonstrated. Avolio and colleagues have shown that, in the Chinese and Australian populations, the observed increase in pulse-wave velocity with age is identical in hypo-, normo-, and hypercholesterolemic patients.[1] In other studies, however, increased rigidity of the aortic wall has been observed in subgroups of hypercholesterolemic subjects.[100] Furthermore, multiple regression analysis in populations of normotensive and hypertensive subjects with or without advanced renal failure indicate a small but significant influence of HDL cholesterol on pulse-wave velocity.[12]

Increased plasma glucose and insulin

For many years, diabetes has been observed to be often but not constantly associated with an increased rigidity of the arterial wall, even at an early phase in asymptomatic patients.[101–103] On the other hand, ambulatory blood pressure measurements reveal that the increase in blood pressure observed in hyperglycemic subjects is principally due to an increase in systolic and pulse pressure.[97] In recent years, however, there was no further development in this research, and the contribution of insulin to arterial rigidity has not yet been extensively evaluated.

Calcifications and abnormalities of the calcium metabolism

Calcifications of the arterial system are observed in several clinical situations involving aging, hypertension, and atherosclerosis. Theoretically, calcifications should greatly contribute to the increased rigidity of the arteries. However, because their size and their number may greatly differ from one subject to another, this contribution remains difficult to evaluate quantitatively. London and colleagues[12,104,105] showed that the role of calcifications on aortic rigidity was modest in a population of normotensive and hypertensive subjects of middle age. In contrast, arterial calcium deposits may contribute substantially to the increased arterial stiffness observed in hypertensive patients undergoing hemodialysis.

In hemodialyzed patients, systolic hypertension is commonly observed in subjects treated for many years by this procedure.[12,22] Aortic cross-sectional area is markedly increased and calcifications may be observed in the overall arterial system, probably related to the well-known disorders of the calcium metabolism observed in such subjects. Based on pulse-wave velocity measurements, aortic rigidity is strikingly increased, and this increase contributes to the development of cardiac hypertrophy through an increase in wave reflections. Drug treatment—particularly calcium-entry blockers—may improve arterial stiffness independently of blood pressure changes.[104] In rats, experimental models involving vitamin D excess and nicotine are able to mimic some of the arterial changes observed in dialyzed patients (see review in reference 105). Such an hemodynamic pattern may play an important role in the increased cardiovascular morbidity and mortality observed in subjects undergoing hemodialysis in the long term.

METABOLIC DISORDERS FOLLOWING DRUG THERAPY FOR HYPERTENSION

It has been widely reported that antihypertensive therapy may induce or favor metabolic disorders, particularly those related to glucose and lipid metabolism.[106,107] Whereas ACE inhibitors, calcium entry blockers, nitrates, and alpha blocking agents cause minor changes in plasma lipids, plasma glucose and insulin resistance, intermediate to major changes are observed following thiazide diuretics and some beta-blocking agents. From this well-admitted classification, it appears that agents causing greater disturbances in glucose and lipid metabolism—diuretics and beta-blocking agents—may cause lesser decrease in arterial rigidity following drug treatment for hypertension (see Table 5-1). Recently, Asmar and colleagues[108] showed that, whereas in hypertensive subjects without drug treatment, pulse-wave velocity was influenced exclusively by age and blood pressure, in treated hypertensive subjects well controlled by drug therapy, pulse-wave velocity was influenced by three independent factors: age, blood pressure, and total-plasma cholesterol. Such an observation indicates that metabolic disorders could influence much more arterial stiffness in the presence than in the absence of antihypertensive therapy.

ATHEROSCLEROSIS AND INCREASED ARTERIAL STIFFNESS

In hypertension and in the aging process, structural and functional changes of the vessels involve the totality of the arterial system, principally the aorta and its major branches. Thus, both aging and hypertension have a great impact on the global level of arterial stiffness. In contrast, atherosclerosis is a more heterogeneous disease and predominates over some particular arteries—for example, the coronary arteries—and more specifically at arterial bifurcations. On these vessels, nonfibrous, and noncalcified plaques do not contribute greatly to an increase in arterial rigidity. However, the atherosclerosis process contributes to the increase of collagen content and calcifications of the vessels and, in the presence of advanced age and/or hypertension, may favor enhanced arterial rigidity.

In clinical medicine, the most important example is given by atherosclerosis of the lower limbs.[109] Increased systolic and pulse pressure are commonly observed in these patients and are due to increased arterial rigidity and wave reflections. Whereas ventricular ejection and vascular resistance are within the normal range, systemic and forearm arterial compliance have been found to be reduced for the same mean arterial pressure as controls. Increased arterial stiffness is exaggerated by high sodium intake and by acute nonselective beta blockade by propranolol. In subjects with atherosclerosis of the lower limbs, increased pulse and systolic pressure are significantly and independently associated with the reduction in the vasodilating properties of the diseased limbs, whereas no comparable association is observed with mean arterial pressure.

In populations of subjects with coronary ischemic disease, no increased incidence of elevated systolic and pulse pressure has been reported. Probably the changes in cardiac function secondary to heart disease contribute to minimize the changes in systolic blood pressure through a decrease in ventricular ejection. Nevertheless, coronary ischemic disease has been found to be significantly associated with reduced aortic compliance.[110] This hemodynamic pattern may contribute to decreased aortic diastolic blood pressure at any given value of mean arterial pressure and therefore to reduce coronary perfusion. Experimentally, decreased aortic compliance exacerbates myocardial ischemia in the presence of stenosis of the coronary artery.[111] Whether this particular mechanism may contribute to the incidence of coronary heart disease following antihypertensive drug therapy is an unresolved question.

Stenosis of the internal carotid artery is associated with an elevated incidence of systolic hypertension.[112] Atherosclerosis of the common carotid artery and of the carotid bifurcation is a classical feature in subjects with essential hypertension, particularly in those over 50 years of age.[59,60] Decreased carotid distensibility is observed in uncomplicated hypertensive subjects for the same age as for normotensive controls.[95] However, the relevance of these abnormalities within the framework of hypertension and atherosclerosis remains to be explored.

Finally, this review shows that many aspects of the clinical management and the pathophysiology of hypertension may be better understood when the status of the large arteries is taken into consideration. Large arteries are not passive conduits; they have an important place in the definition of, the mechanism of, and the therapeutic approach to hypertensive vascular disease.

CONCLUSION

THE ARTERIAL SYSTEM AND
THE THERAPEUTIC TRIALS
OF HYPERTENSION

As we mentioned earlier, many therapeutic trials have been performed in recent years to determine the effectiveness of antihypertensive therapy. Meta-analyses have identified the fact that although the incidences of stroke and congestive heart failure were substantially reduced by antihypertensive drug treatment, the incidences of coronary heart disease were less affected by this treatment, particularly in the younger portion of the population.[66,113] To understand the lack of improvement of coronary ischemic disease, many critical analyses have been performed on various methodological aspects of therapeutic trials. However, there was no study in which it was shown that the basic assumptions of the therapeutic trials themselves may have influenced the quality of their results. Indeed, diastolic blood pressure, and not systolic blood pressure, was the unique criterion of entry. On the other hand, the morbid events evaluated in therapeutic trials are predominantly related to disturbances of the large arteries of the brain, the heart, and the kidney. In this last part of the book, we identify one of the most important biases of therapeutic trials, namely, the dismissal of the problem of the hypertensive large arteries in the definition of hypertension.

BASIC ASSUMPTIONS OF THERAPEUTIC TRIALS AND HYPERTENSIVE
LARGE ARTERIES: A CRITICAL REVIEW

The basis of all therapeutic trials are principally related to blood pressure measurements, which are a key point for any interpretation of anti-hypertensive drug treatment. In this book, we have already noticed several irrelevant but classical assumptions for blood pressure measurements:

- brachial blood pressure is a good index for evaluating systemic blood pressure: this is true for mean blood pressure but not for systolic and diastolic blood pressure, which differ greatly from central to peripheral arteries.
- Increased blood pressure in hypertension is principally characterized by an increase in diastolic blood pressure, a parameter that is directly related to increased vascular resistance. This assumption is untrue, as we showed in the introductory chapter of this book. The reproducibility of systolic blood pressure is much better than that of diastolic blood pressure, and together, both pressures are related to vascular resistance and to arterial compliance.
- Brachial diastolic blood pressure measurements are universally accepted markers for evaluating the results of therapeutic trials after sophisticated statistical evaluations have been performed. The use of these markers for this purpose is obviously not meaningful, because the results of statistical evaluations will be different if blood pressure was measured in other compartments of the arterial tree or if ambulatory blood pressure measurements were performed in place of occasional measurements.

Nevertheless, in this chapter we will limit the discussion to the two most important biases of the therapeutic trials: (i) the curve relating cardiovascular risk to blood pressure level, and (ii) the use of diastolic blood pressure as a criterion of entry for therapeutic trials.

The Curve Relating Cardiovascular Risk to Blood Pressure Level

For epidemiologic studies, three relevant hypothetical models relating cardiovascular risk to blood pressure level have been outlined.[114] These models, which are indicated in Figure 8-1, are analyzed here for a better understanding of the findings of therapeutic trials.

When the relationship between cardiovascular risk and blood pressure is linear and has a high correlation coefficient, then the greater the reduction in risk factors, the lower the risk of disease (Fig. 8-1, curve A). This hypothesis is often assumed in therapeutic trials on hypertension and seems to be especially true from life insurance actuarial data. However, although it seems likely that the curve relating cardiovascular risk to blood pressure is linear above 100 mm Hg diastolic pressures, linearity cannot be completely assumed below this value due to the methodological difficulties in adequately evaluating blood pressure. Furthermore, biologic phenomena are in general not purely linear. With this consideration in mind, it is wise to investigate the possibility that other models, such as those postulating a curvilinear or a

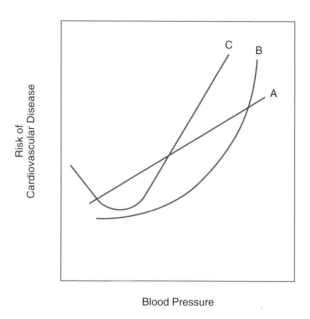

FIGURE 8-1. Three models (A, linear; B, curvilinear; C, U- or J-shaped curve) of hypothetical relationships between risk factors (elevated blood pressure) and risk of cardiovascular disease.

J- or U-shaped relationship, may better explain the role of cardiovascular risk factors on morbidity and mortality.

If the relationship is curvilinear (Fig. 8-1, curve B), the risk decreases with the lowering of blood pressure, but little decrease in the risk of disease can be expected once it has been reduced to the flat part of the curve. In the International Prospective Primary Prevention Study in Hypertension,[115] for instance, the incidence of cardiac events and stroke was found to be positively related to diastolic blood pressure during antihypertensive treatment, but a flatter curve was observed for diastolic pressure below 105 mm Hg. This observation is also corroborated for strokes by the Medical Research Council study,[116] in which only patients with diastolic pressure in the range of 90 to 109 mm Hg were analyzed. The incidence of stroke was significantly reduced in patients randomly assigned to receive antihypertensive agents. However, the benefit of treatment was relatively small: if 850 people with mild hypertension were given antihypertensive drugs for a year, only one stroke would be prevented. Thus, it appears clear that in the lower blood pressure ranges, the cardiovascular risk is small as it relates to the level of blood pressure and its treatment. This finding suggests that factors other than blood pressure itself may be implicated in cardiovascular morbidity and mortality.

Many studies have more recently established that mortality from heart attack is related to diastolic blood pressure in a J-curve, with increased mortality at low as well as at high pressures (Fig. 8-1, curve C). This finding has been observed in untreated as well as in treated patients, and a similar phenomenon has been found in large population studies. Cruickshank and colleagues[117] looked retrospectively at the mortality from myocardial infarction in a study based on 902 consecutive patients attending the hypertension clinic. They found that whereas most attenders had a positive relationship between diastolic blood pressure and heart attack mortality (the lower the pressure, the lower the incidence), in the subgroup of patients with preexisting ischemic heart disease, the curve was J-shaped, with an increase in mortality for achieved diastolic blood pressure below 85 mm Hg. Interestingly, the heart attack mortality versus systolic pressure curve was not a J-curve. Although the numbers of patients in the subgroups were small in this study, the existence of a J-curve was confirmed in several other retrospective analyses.[118] This conceptual approach is important to consider for the interpretation of therapeutic trials but is limited by the fact that brachial diastolic blood pressure and coronary diastolic blood pressure are not equal and have, in fact, quite different values.

Finally, whatever the described epidemiologic model—curvilinear or J-curve—may be, these models are compatible with the possibility that the decrease in diastolic blood pressure following antihypertensive therapy was generated not only by a decrease in vascular resistance but also by a lack of increase (or even a decrease) in aortic compliance at any given value of mean arterial pressure. More specifically, decreased aortic compliance in hypertension may be the mechanism by which a specific fall in diastolic blood pressure occurs at the site of the coronary circulation, a point that was not fully discussed in the various therapeutic trials of hypertension and cannot be recognized from brachial blood pressure measurements.

The Criteria of Entry and Effectiveness of Treatment as a Key Point for the Interpretation of Therapeutic Trials

According to the World Health Organization, sustained hypertension is defined as systolic pressure above 160 mm Hg, diastolic pressure above 95 mm Hg, or both. Despite this definition, in most clinical trials of antihypertensive therapy in the literature, diastolic blood pressure (above 95 mm Hg) was used as the unique criterion for referring hypertensive patients to different primary prevention studies, and systolic blood pressure was not taken into consideration. However, this approach may have greatly modified the interpretation of results, particularly in aged populations, in which intra-arterial brachial diastolic blood pressure is overestimated by cuff pressure measurements.[119]

As an example, Table 8-1 shows the blood pressure levels in patients with hypertension at the time of their entry into the Hypertension Detection Follow-up Program.[120] Patients were divided into three subgroups according to the level of diastolic blood pressure *(DBP)*. In group 1, the diastolic pressure range was 90 to 104 mm Hg. In fact, in this category, it appears clear from Table 6-1 that systolic and pulse pressures were much more elevated than diastolic pressure itself, especially in older patients. In addition, the ratio between pulse pressure *(PP)* and mean arterial pressure *(MBP)* (which may be approximated from the ratio between pulse pressure and diastolic blood pressure because $MBP = DBP + \frac{1}{3} PP$) remains quite similar from group 1 to group 3, but greatly increases with age, pointing to the increasing contribution of pulse and systolic pressures to the manometric definition of hypertension as a function of the aging process (Table 8-1).

According to these observations, it seems likely that the use of diastolic pressure as the exclusive criterion for determining the severity of hypertension may have been prejudicial in the interpretation of therapeutic trials. This important aspect should be recognized both at the entry and at the end of therapeutic trials.

- At the entry of therapeutic trials: in the classical definition of hypertension, elevated systolic and mean arterial pressure may be associated with decreased diastolic pressure, a possibility that was not considered in therapeutic trials; this led to the exclusion of hypertensive patients in the general population who were at particular risk for cardiac hypertrophy and who had altered coronary perfusion (due to altered arterial stiffness). Furthermore, according to the low initial value, it is within the population with the major increase of arterial stiffness in which the best results of therapeutic trials may be expected. In this context, the Systolic Hypertension in the Elderly Program (SHEP)[121] included exclusively elderly subjects with isolated systolic hypertension, a population in which both cardiac and cerebral events are particularly frequent. It is only within this trial that there was a significant decreased incidence of stroke *and* coronary ischemic disease, in agreement with the well-established low of initial value.
- At the end of the therapeutic trials: an important aspect of therapeutic trials was that the level of systolic blood pressure was not taken into account in evaluating the effectiveness of drug therapy, although increased systolic and pulse pressures are more important independent risk factors than diastolic pressure in patients over the age of 50. Subsequently, the characteristics of two different categories of patients have been dismissed following long-term therapeutic trials: those with well-controlled systolic and diastolic blood pressure and those with controlled diastolic blood pressure but with uncontrolled systolic pressure.[122] The

TABLE 8-1. *Systolic and pulse pressure according to level of diastolic pressure at different age ranges in the hypertension Detection and Follow-up Program study*

Pressure	Age (Yrs)	Group 1 (90–104 mm Hg) Medication		Group 2 (90–114 mm Hg) Medication		Group 3 (115+ mm Hg) Medication	
		Yes	No	Yes	No	Yes	No
Diastolic arterial pressure (mm Hg)	30–39	95.0	93.4	102.3	102.6	113.0	116.8
	40–49	94.7	94.2	102.9	102.0	113.4	116.7
	50–59	94.1	94.3	103.4	102.9	114.1	113.8
	60–69	94.4	93.8	102.8	102.3	113.4	113.4
Systolic arterial pressure (mm Hg)	30–39	139.1	136.8	148.0	148.7	163.6	172.0
	40–49	144.0	141.4	156.6	153.2	171.0	176.4
	50–59	149.5	149.1	164.1	163.0	181.6	181.4
	60–69	158.4	158.2	171.0	172.0	189.1	193.3
Pulse pressure (mm Hg)	30–39	44.1	43.4	45.7	46.1	56.6	55.2
	40–49	49.3	47.2	52.7	51.1	57.6	59.7
	50–59	55.1	54.8	60.7	60.2	66.5	67.6
	60–69	64.0	64.4	68.2	69.7	75.7	79.9

Patients were divided into groups according to the level of diastolic blood pressure: the range in group 1 was 90–104 mm Hg; that in group 2, 90–114 mm Hg; and that in group 3, 115 mm Hg or greater. Note that at any level of diastolic pressure, a disproportionate increase in systolic pressure is more frequent above rather than below 50 years.
Mean values are given for each population.
Data from Polt et al.[120]

latter have been shown to be characterized by a more reduced aortic distensibility and a higher degree of cardiac hypertrophy. The prevalence of these patients increases markedly with aging.

Finally, the problem of the large arteries and aortic compliance was largely dismissed in therapeutic trials of hypertension, making the interpretation of the data difficult for two reasons. On the one hand, diuretics, dihydralazine, and β-blocking agents, which have been mostly used in therapeutic trials, are known to cause little modifications in arterial stiffness, despite an adequate blood pressure reduction. On the other hand, with treatment of long duration, the physiologic decrease in aortic compliance with age is not modified by drug treatment and may contribute to decrease *per se* diastolic blood pressure, whereas systolic blood pressure remains elevated. Last, as we already mentioned, in hypertensive subjects, metabolic abnormalities are frequently associated with increased arterial stiffness independent of age and blood pressure and may also complicate the interpretation of the results.

UNANSWERED QUESTIONS RELATED TO THE ROLE OF THE ARTERIES IN THE TREATMENT OF HYPERTENSION

Because arteries were not taken into account in therapeutic trials, several problems now arise in the field of clinical hypertension. In conclusion to this book, some of them are analyzed here.

The Reduction of Cardiovascular Morbidity: Pressure Effect or Drug Effect on the Arterial Tree

One of the basic assumptions of therapeutic trials is that blood pressure reduction is the mechanical factor responsible for decreased morbidity and mortality. However, in such studies, the correlation between the decrease in pressure and the decrease in morbidity was either absent or not published. Even some therapeutic trials showed that the drug effect may be even more important than the pressure effect on the reduction of morbid events.[121] This aspect was particularly shown for diuretics in the MRC trials[123] and in the SHEP study.[121] Thus, diuretics used by the elderly will be taken here as an example to discuss this controversial aspect of drug therapy for hypertension.

In the SHEP study,[121] the criterion of entry in the trial was above normal systolic pressure, with diastolic blood pressure in the normal or low range. Following treatment, there was indeed a decrease in systolic blood pressure but also diastolic blood pressure was lowered. According to the classical WHO definitions of hypertension, normalization of blood pressure by treatment should indeed include a decrease in systolic blood pressure, but diastolic blood pressure should be either maintained or even increased. For that reason, if the classical WHO criterions of hypertension are accepted, the blood pressure profile at the end of the SHEP trial is even better in the placebo group than in the treated group. Indeed, in the former, systolic blood pressure decreased substantially (less than in the treated group), but diastolic blood pressure was maintained. From this simple observation arises the problem of evaluating whether the decreased cardiovascular morbidity in the treated group of the SHEP study was really due to the blood pressure reduction or *to a drug effect on the arterial wall* or to a combination of both factors. Indeed, on the basis of the statistical analysis of the SHEP study, there was no absolute evidence that the reduction of stroke was really due to the decrease in blood pressure alone.

During recent years, the important experimental works of Tobian[124] showed that the incidence of strokes in Stroke-Prone Rats was related to increased sodium intake rather than to elevated blood pressure and that increased sodium intake was associated with strong structural changes of the arteries. In hypertensive humans, we have identified that sodium has a direct effect on arterial diameter and stiffening independently of blood pressure changes.[125] Much more, in the elderly, the reduction of cardiovascular morbidity by diuretics can be partly explained by factors unrelated to control of hypertension, namely, the improvement of subclinical cardiac failure. Finally, it is important to recognize that the clinical pharmacology of diuretics in the field of hypertension is largely unknown. Diuretics were commercialized in hypertension at a period (1960–70) in which clinical pharmacology was not yet developed and during which sodium and renal changes were the quasiexclusive factors taken into account in the mechanisms of action of diuretics. Much remains to be done to fully investigate the effect—independently of the antihypertensive effect—of diuretic compounds (and other antihypertensive agents) on arteries and veins.

At What Age Should Hypertension Be Treated?

From the analysis of therapeutic trials of hypertension, it appears clearly that drug treatment is effective for reducing cardiovascular morbidity, that is, to prevent the complications (the "events") of the disease. In this context, the treatment is much more effective for reducing cardiovascular morbidity in older subjects than it is in younger subjects. Indeed, the reduction of stroke in the elderly trials is the same in percent as in younger populations, but the absolute number is much more important in the older population. In other words, because in the younger population, particularly those below 50 years, the incidence of stroke related to hypertension is extremely low in clinical practice, and because the treatment has minor effects on ischemic coronary disease, the question arises as to whether it is relevant to treat *very early* mild to moderate hypertension in the younger population. In fact, in the previously published classical trials, the age range of the populations was very wide and age was not defined as a critical criterion for entry. Consequently, there is no adequate response to the question: at what age should hypertension be treated?

In terms of pathophysiology of hypertension, it is now common to focus clinical research on the structural cardiovascular changes associated in hypertension. Accordingly, it is believed that hypertension should be treated very early—not only to decrease blood pressure but also to prevent structural changes in the cardiovascular system. It is important to recognize that this question cannot be resolved from studies in animal hypertension, in which there is no epidemiologic aspect of the disease. Furthermore, both in animal and human hypertension, only the structural changes of the heart have been widely studied, although most of the structural changes possibly responsible for cardiovascular morbidity in hypertension are known to occur in the large arterial vessels.

Taken together, these observations suggest that: (i) we know perfectly well that we have to treat the older population, because there is a clear *absolute* benefit in terms of cardiovascular morbidity (that is, in terms of "events"), but (ii) there is no clear evidence from the trials done in the recent years that the same benefit may be obtained in the asymptomatic young population of mild hypertensive subjects, in which strokes occur only above 50 years. In this category of subjects, the interest of prevention of atherosclerosis should be demonstrated.

Of course, the problem of severe, malignant, and secondary hypertension is obviously excluded from this discussion.

What Are the Mechanical Factors Responsible for the Worsening of the Arterial Wall in Hypertension?

For the first time, therapeutic trials in the elderly demonstrated that cardiovascular morbidity was improved in a variety of hypertension that is quite different from that of systolic-diastolic hypertension in middle age: isolated systolic hypertension. Subsequently, the problem is now to investigate whether systolic-diastolic hypertension and isolated systolic hypertension differ in the mechanism by which they may worsen the arterial wall.

We have identified that the arterial wall may be altered through various pressure mechanisms involving increased steady stress, increased pulsatile stress, or even increased variability of these different stresses. Therapeutic trials in hypertension have identified that the change in steady stress (here, by extension, we refer to mean arterial pressure) may improve cardiovascular morbidity and mortality, particularly in sustained systolic–diastolic hypertension of the middle-age. However, studies of hypertension in the elderly indicate that pulsatile stress and its variability might be the predominant hemodynamic factor altering the arterial wall in this category of patient. Thus, it appears that different forms of tensiles stresses may affect the arterial wall and, consequently, cardiovascular morbidity.

In this book, the analysis of the mechanical factors altering the arterial wall was limited to tensile stress. Also, blood flow, through shear stress, may affect the arterial wall in hypertension. Today, in the field of clinical hypertension, in vivo evaluation of tensile and shear stresses as principal worsening factors acting on the arterial wall is one of the principal challenges in cardiovascular research.

REFERENCES

1. Nichols WV, O'Rourke MF. *McDonald's Blood Flow in Arteries: Theoretical, Experimental and Clinical Principles*, 3rd ed. London, Melbourne, Auckland: Edward Arnold, 1990;77–142, 216–269, 283–269, 398–437.
2. Safar ME. Pulse pressure in essential hypertension: clinical and therapeutical implications *J Hypertension*. 1989;7:768–776.
3. Dobrin PB. Vascular mechanics. In: Sheperd JT, Abboud FM, eds. Geiger SR, exec. ed. *Handbook of Physiology. Section 2: The Cardiovascular System. Volume III. Peripheral Circulation and Organ Blood Flow, Part I*. Bethesda, Maryland: American Physiological Society, 1983;65–102.
4. Dobrin PB, Mrkvicka R. Estimating the elastic modulus of non-atherosclerotic elastic arteries. *J Hypertension*. 1992;10(suppl 6) S7–S10.
5. Cox RH. Basis for the altered arterial wall mechanics in the spontaneously hypertensive rat. *Hypertension*. 1981;3:485–495.
6. Safar ME, Levy BI, Laurent S, London GM. Hypertension and the arterial system: clinical and therapeutic aspects. *J Hypertension*. 1990;8(suppl 7):S113–S119.
7. Pohl U, Holtz J, Busse R, Bassenge E. Crucial role of endothelium in the vasodilator response to increased flow in vivo. *Hypertension*. 1986;8:37–44.
8. Laurent S, Lacolley P, Brunel P, Laloux B, Safar ME. Flow-dependent vasodilation of brachial artery in essential hypertension. *Am J Physiol*. 1990;258(*Heart Circ. Physiol.*):27:H1004–H1011.
9. Kelly R, Hayward C, Ganis J, Daley J, Avolio A, O'Rourke M. Noninvasive determination of age-related changes in the human arterial pulse. *Circulation*. 1989;80:1652–1659.
10. Kelly RP. Pharmacological potential for reversing the ill effects of ageing and of arterial hypertension in central aortic systolic pressure. *J Hypertension*. 1992;10(suppl 6):S97–S100.
11. Benetos A, Tsoucaris-Kupfer D, Favereau X, Corcos T, Safar M. Carotid artery tonometry: an accurate non-invasive method for central aortic pulse pressure evaluation. *J Hypertension*. 1991;9(suppl 6):S144–S145.
12. London GM, Marchais SJ, Safar ME, Genest AF, Guerin AP, Metivier F, Chedid K, and London AM. Aortic and large artery compliance in end-stage renal failure. *Kidney International*. 1990;37:137–142.

13. London GM, Guerin AP, Pannier BM, Marchais SJ, and Metivier F. Body height as a determinant of carotid pulse contour in humans; *J Hypertension*. 1992;1(suppl 6):S93–S96.

14. Tsoucaris-Kupfer D, Benetos A, Legrand M, Safar M. Pulse pressure gradient along the aortic tree in normotensive Wistar-Kyoto and spontaneously hypertensive rats: effect of nicardipine. *J Hypertension*. 1993;11:135–139.

15. Hugue CJ, Safar ME, Aliefierakis MC, Asmar RG, London GM. The ratio between ankle and brachial systolic pressure in patients with sustained uncomplicated essential hypertension. *Clin Sci* 1988;74:179–182.

16. Kannel WB, Stokes JLL. Hypertension as a cardiovascular risk factor. In: Bulpitt CJ, ed. *Handbook of Hypertension, IV, Epidemiology of Hypertension*. Amsterdam: Elsevier Science; 1985:15–34.

17. Kannel WB, Gordon T, Schwartz MJ. Systolic versus diastolic blood pressure and risk of coronary heart disease: The Framingham Study. *Am J Cardiol*. 1971; 27:335–346.

18. Darné B, Girerd X, Safar ME, Cambien F, Guize L. Pulsatile versus steady component of blood pressure: A cross-sectional and a prospective analysis on cardiovascular mortality. *Hypertension*. 1989;13:392–400.

19. Pannier B, Brunel P, El Aroussy W, Lacolley P, and Safar ME. Pulse pressure and echocardiographic findings in essential hypertension. *J Hypertension*. 1989; 7:127–132.

20. Latham RD. Pulse propagation in the systemic arterial tree. In: Westerhof N, Gross DR, eds. *Vascular Dynamics: Physiological perspectives*. New York and London: Plenum Press, 1989:49–68.

21. Labouret G, Achimastos A, Benetos A, Safar M, Housset E. L'hypertension artérielle systolique des amputés traumatiques. *Press Med*. 1983;21:1349–1354.

22. London GM, Guerin AP, Pannier B, Marchais SJ, Metivier F, Safar ME. Arterial wave reflections and increased systolic and pulse pressure in chronic uremia: Study using noninvasive carotid pulse waveform registration.*Hypertension*. 1992;20:10–19.

23. Murgo JP, Westerhof N, Giolma JP, Altobelli SA. Aortic input impedance in normal man; relationship to pressure shapes. *Circulation*. 1980;62:105–116.

24. Marchais SJ, Guerin AP, Pannier BM, Levy BI, Safar ME, London GM. Wave reflections and cardiac hypertrophy in chronic uremia. *Hypertension*. 1993;22: 876–883.

25. Latson TW, Hunter WC, Katoh N, Sagawa K. Effect of nitroglycerin on aortic impedance, diameter and pulse wave velocity. *Circ Res*. 1988;62:884–880.

26. Yaginuma T, Avolio AP, O'Rourke MF, Nichols WW, Morgan J, Roy P, Baron D, Branson J, Feneley M. Effect of glyceryl trinitrate on peripheral arteries alters left ventricular hydraulic load in man. *Cardiovasc Res*. 1986;20:153–60.

27. Safar ME. Antihypertensive effects of nitrates in chronic human hypertension . *J of Appl Cardiol*. 1990,5:69–81.

28. Laurent S, Arcaro G, Benetos A, Lafleche A, Hoeks A, Safar ME. Mechanism of nitrate-induced improvement on arterial compliance depends on vascular territory. *J Cardiovasc Pharmacol*. 1992; 19:641–649.

29. Taylor MG. Wave travel in arteries and the design of the cardiovascular system. In: Attinger EO, ed. *Pulsatile Blood Flow*. New York: Mc Graw Hill; 1964:343–347.

30. Safar ME, Peronneau PA, Levenson JA, Toto-Moukouo JA, Simon A Ch. Pulsed Doppler: Diameter, Blood flow velocity and volumic flow of the brachial artery in sustained essential hypertension. *Circulation*. 1981;63:393–399.

31. Isnard RN, Pannier BM, Laurent S, London GM, Diebold B, Safar ME. Pulsatile diameter and elastic modulus of the aortic arch in essential hypertension: a non-invasive study. *J Am Coll Cardiol*. 1989;13:399–405.

32. Hoeks APG, Brands PJ, Smeets GAM, Reneman RS. Assessment of the distensibility of superficial arteries. *Ultrasound Med Biol*. 1990;16:121–128.

33. Tardy Y, Meister JJ, Perret F, Waeber B, Brunner HR. Assessment of the elastic behaviour of peripheral arteries from a non-invasive measurement of theirs diameter-pressure curves. *Clin Phys Physiol Meas*. 1991:12:39–54.

34. Kawasaki T, Sasayama S, Yagi SI, Asakawa T, Hirai T. Non-Invasive assessment of the age related changes in stiffness of the human arteries. *Cardiovasc Res*. 1987;21:678–687.

35. Laurent S. Arterial wall hypertrophy and stiffness in essential hypertensive patients. *J Hypertension*.1995;26:355–362.

36. Boutouyrie P, Laurent S, Benetos A, Girerd X, Hoeks APG, Safar ME. Opposite effects of ageing on distal and proximal large arteries in hypertensives. *J Hypertension*.1992;10(suppl 6):S87–S92.

37. Linder L, Kiowski W, Buhler FR, Lüscher TF. Indirect evidence for release of endothelium-derived relaxing factor in human forearm circulation in vivo: blunted response in essential hypertension. *Circulation*. 1990;81:1762–1767.

38. Panza JA, Quyyumi AA, Brush JE,Epstein SE . Abnormal endothelium-dependent vascular relaxation in patients with essential hypertension. *N Engl J Med*. 1990;323:22–27.

39. Milnor WR. *Hemodynamics*. Baltimore/London: Williams & Wilkins, 1982:56–96.

40. Liu Z, Ting C-T, Zhu S, Yin FCP. Aortic compliance in human hypertension. *Hypertension*. 1989;140:129–136.

41. Finkelstein SM, Collins VR, Cohn JN. Arterial vascular compliance response to vasodilators by Fourier and pulse contour analysis. *Hypertension*.1988;12:380–387.

42. Levy BI, Michel JB, Salzmann JL, Azizi M, Poitevin F, Safar ME, Camilleri JP. Effects of chronic inhibition of converting enzyme on mechanical and structural properties of arteries in rat renovascular hypertension. *Circ Res*. 1988;63:227–229.

43. Yin FCP and Zharong Liu. Arterial compliance-physiological viewpoint. In: Westerhof N, Gross, DR, eds. *Vascular Dynamics: Physiological perspectives*. New York and London: Plenum Press, 1989:9–22.

44. Simon AC, Safar ME, Levenson JA, London M, Levy BI, Chau NP. An evaluation of large arteries compliance in man. *Am J Physiol*. 1979;237:H550–H556.

45. Ting CE, Brin KP, Lin SJ, Wang SP, Chang MS, Chiang BN, Yin FCP. Arterial hemodynamics in human hypertension. *J Clin Invest*. 1986;78:1462–1473.

46. Levy BI, Babalis D, Lacolley P, Poitevin P, Safar ME. Cardiac hypertrophy and characteristic impedance in spontaneously hypertensive rats. *J Hypertension*. 1988;(suppl 4):S110–S111.

47. Simon AC, Laurent S, Levenson J, Bouthier J, Safar M. Estimation of forearm arterial compliance in normal and hypertensive men from simultaneous pressure and flow measurements in the brachial artery, using a pulsed Doppler device and a first-order arterial model during diastole. *Cardiovasc Res*. 1983;17:331–338.

48. Gribbin B, Pickering TG, Sleight P. Arterial distensibility in normal and hypertensive man. *Clin Sci.* 1979;56:413–417;

49. Avolio AP, Deng FQ, Li WQ, Luo YF, Huang ZD, Xing LF, O'Rourke MF. Effects on aging on arterial distensibility in populations with high and low prevalence of hypertension: comparison between urban and rural communities in China. *Circulation.* 1985;71:202–215.

50. Smulyan H, Vardan S, Griffiths A, Gribbin B. Forearm arterial distensibility in systolic hypertension. *J Am Coll Cardiol.* 1984;3:387–394.

51. Girerd X, Chanudet X, Larroque P, Clement R, Laloux B, Safar ME. Early arterial modifications in young patients with borderline hypertension. *J Hypertension.* 1989;7(suppl 1):S45–S47.

52. Safar ME, Laurent S, Pannier BM, London GM. Structural and functional modifications of peripheral large arteries in hypertensive patients, *J Clin Hypertension.* 1987;3:360–367.

53. Benetos A, Laurent S, Hoeks AP, Boutouyrie PH, Safar ME. Arterial alterations with ageing and high blood pressure: a non-invasive study of carotid and femoral arteries. *Arteriosclerosis Thrombosis.* 1993;13:90–97.

54. Boutouyrie P, Lacolley P, Laurent S, London GM, Safar ME. Intrinsic modifications of the brachial and the radial arteries in hypertensive humans. *Clin Invest Med.* 1994;2:97–106.

55. Hayoz D,Rutschmann B, Perret F, Niederberger M, Tardy Y, Mooser V, Nussberger J, Waeber B, Brunner H. Conduit artery compliance and distensibility are not necessarily reduced in hypertension. *Hypertension.* 1992;20:1–6.

56. Yin FCP. The aging vasculature and its effects on the heart. In: Weisfeldt ML, ed. *The Aging Heart (Aging XII)*, chap 7. New York: Raven Press; 1990:137–213.

57. Burton AC. Relation of structure to function of tissues of the wall of blood vessels. *Physiol Rev.* 1954;34:619–642.

58. Dobrin PB, Baker WH, Gley WC. Elastolytic and collagenolytic studies of arteries: implications for the mechanical properties of aneurysms. *Arch Surg.* 1984;119:406–409.

59. Roman MJ, Pini R, Pickering G Th, Devereux R. Non-Invasive measurements of arterial compliance in hypertensive compared with normotensive adults. *J Hypertension.* 1992;10(suppl 6):S115–S118.

60. Bond MG, Wilmoth S.K, Envold GL, Strickland HL. Detection and monitoring of asymptomatic atherosclerosis in clinical trials. *Am J Med.* 1989;86(suppl 4A):33–36.

61. Girerd X, Mourad JJ, Acar C, Heudes D, Chiche S, Bruneval P, Mignot JP, Safar M, Laurent S. Non-invasive measurement of medium sized artery intima-media thickness in humans—in vitro validation. *J. Vasc Res.* 1994;31:114–120.

62. Treasure Ch B, Manoukian SV, Klein JL, Vita JA, Nabel EG, Renwick GH, Selwyn AP, Alexander RW, Ganz P. Epicardial coronary artery responses to acetylcholine are impaired in hypertensive patients. *Circ Res.* 1992;71:776–781.

63. Levy BI, Benessiano J, Poitevin P, Safar ME. Endothelium dependent mechanical properties of the carotid artery in WKY and SHR: role of angiotensin converting enzyme inhibition. *Circ Res.* 1990;66:321–328.

64. Safar ME, Toto-Moukouo JJ, Bouthier JA, Asmar RE, Levenson JA, Simon AC, London GM. Arterial dynamics, cardiac hypertrophy, and antihypertensive treatment. *Circulation.*1987;75(suppl 1):156–161.

65. Glagov S, Vito R, Giddens D P, Zarins Ch K. Micro-architecture and composition of artery walls: relationship to location, diameter and the distribution of mechanical stress. *J Hypertension*. 1992;10(suppl 6):S101–S104.

66. Thomson SG. An appraisal of the large-scale trials of anti-hypertensive treatment. In: Bulpitt CJ. ed. *Epidemiology of Hypertension (Handbook of Hypertension, vol 6)*. Amsterdam: Elsevier, 1985:331–343.

67. Safar ME, Simon AC, Levenson JA, Cazor JL . Hemodynamic effects of diltiazem in hypertension. *Circ Res*. 1983;52 (suppl 1):169–173.

68. Simon AC, Levenson JA, Levy BI, Bouthier JE, Peronneau PP, Safar ME. Effect of nitroglycerin on peripheral large arteries in hypertension *Br J Clin Pharmacol*. 1982;14:241–246.

69. Safar ME, Laurent S, Bouthier JD, London GM, Mimran A. Effect of converting enzyme inhibitors on hypertension large arteries in humans. *Am J Hypertension*. 1986;8:1257–1261.

70. Asmar RG, Pannier B, Santoni JPH, Laurent St, London GM, Levy BI, Safar ME. Reversion of cardiac hypertrophy and reduced arterial compliance after converting enzyme inhibition in essential hypertension. *Circulation*. 1988;78:941–950.

71. O'Rourke, M, Safar ME, Dzau VJ. *Arterial Vasodilation. Mechanisms and Therapy*. London, Melbourne, Auckland: Edward Arnold, 1993:62–101, 149–179.

72. Asmar RG, Journo HJ, Lacolley PJ, Santoni JP, Billaud E, Levy BI, Safar M. Treatment of one year with perindopril: effect on cardiac mass and arterial compliance in essential hypertension. *J Hypertension*. 1988;6(suppl 3):S23–S25.

73. Asmar R, Benetos A, Brahimi M, Chaouche K, Safar M. Arterial and antihypertensive effects of nitrendipine: a double blind comparison versus placebo. *J Cardiovasc Pharmacol*. 1992;20:858–863.

74. Safar ME, Pannier B, Laurent S, London GM. Calcium-entry blockers and arterial compliance in hypertension. *J Cardiovasc Pharmacol*. 1989;14(suppl 10):S1–S6.

75. Masafumi Y, Toshiaki F, Masunori M. Effect of diltiazem on aortic pressure-diameter relationship in dogs. *Am J Physiol*. 1989;256:H1580–H1587.

76. Smulyan H, Mookherjee S, Warner RA. The effect of nitroglycerin on forearm arterial distensibility. *Circulation*. 1986;73:1264–1269.

77. Levenson J, Simon AC, Bouthier JC, Benetos A, Safar ME. Post-synaptic alpha-blockade and brachial artery compliance in essential hypertension. *J Hypertension*. 1984;2:37–41.

78. Levy BI, Benessiano J, Poitevin P, Lukin I, Safar ME. Systemic arterial compliance in normotensive and hypertensive rats. *J Cardiovasc Pharmacol*. 1985;7(suppl):S28–S32.

79. Levy BI, Poitevin P, Safar ME. Effects of alpha-1 adrenoceptor blockade on arterial compliance in normotensive and spontaneously hypertensive rats. *Hypertension*. 1990;17:534–540.

80. Asmar RG, Kerihuel JC, Girerd XJ, Safar ME. Effect of Bisoprolol on blood pressure and arterial hemodynamics in systemic hypertension. *Am J Cardiol*. 1991;68:61–64.

81. De Luca N, Rosiello G, Crispino M, et al. Effects of chronic antihypertensive treatment with ketanserin versus metoprolol on blood pressure and large arteries compliance in humans: a cross-over double-blind study. *J Clin Pharmacol*. 1988;28:332–338.

82. Trimarco B, Lemb G, De Luca N. Effects of celiprolol on systemic and forearm circulation in hypertensive patients: a double-blind cross-over study versus metoprolol . J Clin Pharmacol. 1987;27:593–600.

83. Pithois-Merli IM, Cournot AX, Georges DR, Pappo M, Safar ME. Acute effect of labetalol on hypertensive brachial artery. J Clin Hypertension. 1987;3:479–486.

84. Watkins RW, Sybertz EJ, Atonellis A, Pula K, Rivelli M. Effects of the antihypertensive agent dilevalol on aortic compliance in anesthetized dogs. J Cardiovasc Pharmacol. 1987;12:42–40.

85. Safar ME, Asmar RG, Benetos A, London GM, Levy BI. Sodium, large arteries and diuretic compounds in hypertension. J Hypertension. 1992;10(suppl 6):S133–S136.

86. Asmar RG, Benetos A, Chaouche-Teyara K, Raveau Landon C, Safar M. Comparison of effects of felodipine versus hydrochlorothiazide on arterial diameter and pulse-wave velocity in essential hypertension. Am J Cardiol. 1993;72:794–798.

87. Levy BI, Poitevin P, Safar ME. Effects of indapamide on the mechanical properties of the arterial wall in dexosycorticosterone acetate-salt hypertensive rats. Am J Cardiol. 1990;65:28H–32H.

88. Levy BI, Curmi P, Poitevin P, Safar ME. Modifications of the arterial mechanical properties of normotensive and hypertensive rats without arterial pressure changes. J Cardiovasc Pharmacol. 1989;14:253–259.

89. Simon AC, Levenson J, Bouthier JD, Safar ME. Effects on chronic administration of enalapril and propranolol on the large arteries in essential hypertension. J Cardiovasc Pharmacol. 1985;7:856–861.

90. Bouthier JA, Safar ME,Curien ND,London GM, Levenson JA, Simon AC. Effect of cadralazine on brachial artery hemodynamics and forearm venous tone in essential hypertension. Clin Pharmacol Ther. 1986;39:82–88.

91. Achimastos A, Girerd X, Simon AC, Pithois-Merli I, Levenson J. The efficacy of a transdermal formulation of clonidine in mild to moderate hypertension and its effects on the arterial and venous vasculature of the forearm. Eur J Clin Pharmacol. 1987;33:111–114.

92. Van Merode T, Van Bortel L, Smeets FA, Buhom R, Mooij J, Rahn KH, Reneman RS. The effect of verapamil on carotid artery distensibility and cross-sectional compliance in hypertensive patients. J Cardiovasc Pharmacol. 1990;15:109–103.

92a. Kool MJ, Lusterman FA, Breed JG, Stuyker-Boudier HA, Hoeks AP, Van Bortel LM. Effect of perindopril and amiloride/hydrochlorothiazide on haemodynamics and vessel wall properties of large arteries. J Hypertens. 1995;13:839–848.

93. Sihm I, Schroeder AP, Aalkjaer C, Holm M, Morn B, Mulvany MJ, Thygesen K, Lederballe O. Normalization of resistance artery structure and left ventricular morphology. Can J Cardiol. 1994;10(suppl D): 30D–32D.

93a. Thybo NK, Stephens N, Cooper A, Aalkjer C, Heagerty AM, Mulvany MJ. Effect of antihypertensive treatment on small arteries of patients with previously untreated essential hypertension. Hypertension. 1995; 25(part 1):474-81.

93b. London GM, Pannier B, Guerin A. Marchais SJ, Safar M, Cuche JL. Cardiac hypertrophy, aortic compliance, peripheral resistance, and wave reflection in end-stage renal disease. Comparative effects of ACE inhibition and calcium channel blockade. Circulation. 1994;90:2786–96.

94. Girerd X, Mourad JJ, Copie C et al. Noninvasive detection of an increased vascular mass in untreated hypertensive patients. Am J Hypertens. 1994;7:1076-84.

95. Arcaro G, Laurent S, Jondeau G, Hoeks AP, Safar ME. Stiffness of the common carotid artery in treated hypertensive patients. *J Hypertension*. 1991;9:947–954.

96. Brunel P, Girerd X, Laurent S, Pannier B, Safar M. Acute changes in forearm haemodynamics produced by cigarette smoking in healthy normotensive non-smokers are not influenced by propranolol or pindolol. *Eur J CLin Pharmacol*. 1992;42:143–146.

97. Asmar RG, Girerd XJ, Brahimi M, Safavian A, Safar ME. Ambulatory blood pressure measurement, smoking and abnormalities of glucose and lipid metabolism in essential hypertension. *J Hypertension*. 1992;10:181–187.

98. Henry PD. Inappropriate coronary vasomotion: excessive constriction and insufficient dilation. In: Sperakakis N., ed. *Physiology and pathophysiology of the Heart*. Dordrecht: Kluwer Academic Publishers, 1989:975–991.

99. Creager MA, Gallagher SJ, Girerd XJ, Coleman SM, Dzau VJ, Cooke JP. Arginine improves endothelium-dependent vasodilation in hypercholesterolemic humans. *J Clin Invest*. 1992;90:1248–1253.

100. Relf IRN, Lo CS, Myers KA, Wahlwvist MI. Risk factors for changes in aortic-iliac arterial compliance in healthy men. *Arteriosclerosis*. 1986;6:105–108.

101. Woolam GL, Shner PL, Valbona BS, Hoff HE. The pulse wave velocity as an early indicator of atherosclerosis in diabetic subjects. *Circulation*. 1962;25:533–539.

102. Pillsbury HC, Hung W, Kyle MC, Freis ED. Arterial pulse waves velocity and systolic time intervals in diabetic children. *Am Heart J*. 1974;87:783–790.

103. Scarpello JH, Martin TR, Ward JD. Ultrasound measurements of pulse-wave velocity in the peripheral arterie of diabetic subjects. *Clin Sci*.1980;58:53–57.

104. London GM, Marchais SJ, Guerin AP, Metivier F, Safar ME, Fabiani F, Froment L. Salt and water retention and calcium blockade in uremia. *Circulation*. 1990; 82:105–113.

105. London GM, Safar ME, Levy BI. In: Epstein M, ed. *Calcium Antagonists in Clinical Medicine*. Philadelphia: Hanley and Belfus, Mosby Yearbook; 1992:89–103.

106. Weidmann P, Gerber A, Mordasini R. Effects of antihypertensive therapy on serum lipoproteins. *Hypertension*. 1987;5(suppl 3):120–131.

107. Pollare T, Lithell H, Berne C. A comparison of the effects of hydrochlorothiazide and captopril on glucose and lipid metabolism in patients with hypertension. *N Engl J Med*. 1989;321:868–873.

108. Asmar RG, Hugue CH, London GM, Weiss YW, Laloux BM, Safar ME. Aortic Stiffness in Treated Hypertensive Patients. *Blood Pressure*.1995;4:48–54.

109. Safar ME. Atherosclerotic hypertension: systolic hypertension and arterial compliance in patients with arteriosclerosis obliterans of the lower limbs. In: Safar ME, Fouad Tarazi F, ed. *The Heart in Hypertension*. Dordrecht: Kluwer Academic Publishers; 1989:123–133.

110. Stefanadis C, Wooley CF, Bush CA, Kolibash AJ, Boudoulas J. Aortic distensibility abnormalities in coronary artery disease. *Am J Cardiol*. 1987;59:1300–1304.

111. Watanabe H, Ohtsuka S, Kakihana M, Sugishita Y. Coronary circulation in dogs with an experimental decrease in aortic compliance. *J Am Coll Cardiol*. 1993;21: 1497–1506.

112. Safar ME, Laurent S, Benetos A, London GM. The common carotid circulation in patients with essential hypertension. *Stroke*. 1988;19:1198–1202.

113. Collins R, Peto R, Macmahon S, Hebert P, Fiebach NH, Everlein KA, Godwin J, Quizilbash N, O'Taylor J, Hennekens C. Blood pressure, stroke, and coronary

heart disease: part 2. Short-term reductions in blood pressure: overview of randomized drug trials in their epidemiological context. *Lancet.* 1990;335: 827–838.

114. Safar ME. Therapeutic trials and large arteries in hypertension. *Am Heart J.* 1988;115:702–719.

115. The IPPPSH Collaborative Group. Cardiovascular risk and risk factors in a randomized trial of treatment based on the beta-blocker oxprenolol: the International prospective primary prevention study in hypertension (IPPPSF). *J Hypertension.* 1985;3:379–392.

116. Mial WE. The mild hypertension dilemma: results to the British MRC Trial. *J Clin Hypertension.* 1986;3:12s–21s.

117. Cruickshank JM. Coronary flow reserve and the J curve relation between diastolic blood pressure and myocardial infarction. *Br Med J.* 1988;297:1227–1230.

118. Farnett L, Murrow CD, Linn WD, Lucey CR, Tuley MR. The J-curve phenomenon and the treatment of hypertension: is there a point beyond which pressure reduction is dangerous? *JAMA.* 1990;265:489–495.

119. Safar ME, Laurent ST, Asmar RE, Safavian A, London GM. Systolic hypertension in patients with arteriosclerosis obliterans of the lower limbs. *Angiology.* 1987;28:287–295.

120. Polk FB, Cutter G, Dugherty RM. Hypertension detection and follow-up program: baseline physical examination characteristics of the hypertensive participants. *Hypertension.*1983;5:IV 92–IV 99.

121. SHEP Cooperative Research Group. Prevention of stroke by antihypertensive drug treatment in older persons with isolated systolic hypertension: final results of the Systolic Hypertension in the Elderly program (SHEP). *JAMA.* 1991;265: 3255–3264.

122. Safar ME, Soubies PHL, Safavian AM, Asmar RG, Laurent ST. Antihypertensive therapy with uncontrolled systolic pressure and increased aortic rigidity. In: Omae T., Zanchetti A, eds. *How Should Elderly Hypertensive Patients Be treated ?* New York: Springer Verlag; 1989:143–150.

123. MRC Working Party. Medical Research Council trial of treatment of hypertension in older adults: principal results. *Br Med J.* 1992;304:405–412.

124. Tobian L. Salt and hypertension lessons from animal models that relate to human hypertension. *Hypertension.* 1991;17 (suppl 1):152–158

125. Benetos A, Yang-Yan X, Cuche JL, Hannaert P, Safar M. Arterial effects of salt restriction in hypertensive patients: A 9-week, randomized double-blind, crossover study. *J Hypertension.* 1992;10:355–360.

INDEX

A

Adrenergic blocking agents affecting arterial diameters and compliance, 50, 54–56
Age
and aortic compliance, 81
and blood pressure curve, 6, 63, 64
and changes in larger arteries, 43
and hemodynamics of hypertension, 13
and increased wave reflections, 29–30
and initiation of antihypertensive therapy, 80–81
long-term drug treatment of hypertension in relation to, 63–67
and mechanical properties of arteries, 35
and mismatch between heart and vessels, 27
Peterson elastic modulus in relation to, 63, 64
and pulse pressure measurements, 23–24, 25
and pulse-wave velocity, 37–38, 43
Alpha-adrenoreceptors, arterial effects of, 54–56
Angiotensin converting enzyme (ACE) inhibitors, 50–52
affecting arterial dilation and compliance, 17, 49, 50
affecting wave reflections, 59
Ankle and brachial systolic pressure measurements, 24
Antihypertensive therapy
affecting structural changes in

arteries, 61–63
affecting wave reflections, 30, 58–60
age at initiation of, 80–81
in arterial compliance, 50
effects of, on arterial system, 49–60
effects on arterial tree, 17, 79–80
metabolic disorders after, 69
role of aging process following, 63
stepped care approach in, 63
therapeutic trials in, 75–85
Aorta
age-related changes in, 35, 43
compliance of, 39–40
in coronary artery disease, 72
and coronary perfusion pressure, 25
and diastolic blood pressure, 76, 79
in hypertension, 37
diastolic diameter in hypertension, 33
pulse-wave velocity, 37–38
rigidity affected by calcifications, 69
stiffness of
in hypertension, 44
and pulse pressure increase, 25
wave reflections
related to age, 29
in ventricular hypertrophy, 30
Aortic arch, nitrates affecting, 54
Applanation tonometry, 21–22, 28, 39
Arterial compliance
antihypertensive agents in, 50
calcium blockade modification of, 53

Arterial dilation, causes of, 49
Arterial stiffening, in hypertension, 49
Arterial system
  effects of antihypertensive therapy on, 49–60
  function of, 11–13
  geometric and mechanical properties of, 16–17
  pressure-volume relationship in, 13–16
  sodium- and diuretic-induced changes in, 56–58
  stress-strain relationship in, 17–19
Arterial wall, drug-induced changes in, 50, 53
Arteriolar vasodilator, blood pressure reduction due to, 53
Atenolol
  affecting arterial structure, 61, 62
  affecting wave reflections, 59
Atherosclerosis, arterial stiffness in, 72

B

Beta-adrenoreceptors, arterial action of, 54
Bisoprolol and arterial compliance, 56
Blood flow velocity, nitrates affecting, 54
Blood pressure. *See also* Diastolic blood pressure; Systolic blood pressure
  reduction of, due to arteriolar vasodilators, 53
  verapamil affecting, 52
Blood pressure curve
  age affecting, 6, 63, 64
  Fourier analysis of, 2–4
  pulsatile and steady components of, 3–4
Brachial artery
  adrenergic blocking agents affecting, 54–56
  bisoprolol affecting, 56
  blood pressure measurements, 74

with ankle systolic pressure, 24
cadralazine affecting, 53
calcium channel blockers affecting, 52, 53
compliance and distensibility in, 39–40, 56
diameter and wall motion studies, 31–32
  diastolic diameter in hypertension, 33
  diltiazem and dihydralazine affecting, 49
effects of perindopril on diameter of, 51
hemodynamics in, 56
high flow dilation at site of, 50
mechanical properties in hypertension, 35
nicorandil affecting, 53
nitrates affecting, 54
nitrendipine affecting, 53
norepinephrine affecting, 56
parameters in normotension and hypertension, 42
sodium affecting, 56

C

Cadralazine affecting arterial diameter, 53
Calcifications, and arterial stiffness, 68–69
Calcium channel blockers
  affecting arterial dilation and compliance, 17, 52, 53
  affecting wave reflections, 59
  effects in dialysis patients, 69
Calcium metabolism disorders, arterial stiffness in, 69
Capacitance, 14
Captopril, converting enzyme inhibition by, 51
Cardiac hypertrophy
  perindopril affecting, 62
  reversion of, 62
Cardiac mass increase. *See* Ventricular hypertrophy
Cardiovascular risk and blood pres-

sure levels, 24–25, 74–76
Carotid artery
  age-related changes in, 35, 43
  calcium channel blockers affecting, 52, 53
  compliance and distensibility in, 39–40, 56
  diameter and wall motion studies, 31–32
  diastolic diameter in hypertension, 33
  distensibility in hypertension, 72
  mechanical properties affected by age, 35, 63
  nitrates affecting, 54
  plaque buildup in, 43
  pulse pressure, 23
    in hypertension, 24
    waveform recording of, 28
  wave reflections related to age, 29
Central arteries. *See also* Aorta; Carotid artery
  diameters compared to peripheral arteries, 33–35, 45
  indices in hypertension, 35–40
    in arterial segments, 38–40
    in systemic arteries, 36–38
  metabolic factors and smoking affecting, 67–69
  wall structure in, 45
Cholesterol excess, and arterial stiffness, 68
Circumferential stress, and thickness of arterial wall, 17–18
Collagen
  fiber tension, 15, 16–17
  and mechanical properties of arteries, 41–42
Compliance, 14–15
  aortic
    in coronary artery disease, 72
    and coronary perfusion pressure, 25
    and diastolic blood pressure, 76, 79
    in hypertension, 37
    decrease in elderly, 13
    dilation of arteries affecting,

16–17
  drug therapy affecting, 17
  hypertension affecting, 35
    in arterial segments, 38–40
    in systemic arteries, 36–38
  related to vasodilation, 16–17
Conduit function of arteries, 11
Coronary arteries
  diastolic pressure affected by aortic compliance, 76
  disease after antihypertensive therapy, 72, 75
  factors affecting perfusion pressure, 25
  nitrates affecting, 53–54
Counter-regulatory mechanisms, drug-induced, 49
Cushioning function of arteries, 12

D

Definitions of hypertension, 1–2, 5–6, 76
Diabetes mellitus, arterial stiffness in, 68
Dialysis patients. *See* Renal failure, end-stage
Diameter of arteries
  calcium-entry blockers affecting, 52, 53
  changes in systole and diastole, 18, 34
  diastolic values in hypertension, 33
  increased from flow velocity changes, 17
  sodium-and diuretic-induced changes in, 56–58
Diastole, arterial diameter changes in, 34
Diastolic blood pressure
  age affecting, 63, 67
  aortic compliance affecting, 76, 79
  arterial stiffness affecting, 12
  and cardiovascular risk, 24–25, 75–76
  and coronary perfusion, 25
  in hypertension, 2, 5, 74

Dihydralazine affecting brachial
    artery diameter, 49
Dilevalol affecting wave reflections,
    59
Diltiazem affecting brachial artery
    diameter, 49
Distending pressure, and stress-strain
    relationship, 17–19
Distensibility, 15, 16
    aortic, 39–40
    hypertension affecting, 35
    and measurements of diameter
        changes, 31–33
Diuretics
    affecting arterial diameter, 56–58
    antihypertensive effects of, 79–80
Drug-induced changes
    in arterial wall, 50
    in smooth muscle, 17, 49, 53
    in wave reflections, 30, 58–60
Drug therapy. See Antihypertensive
    therapy

E

Echo-Doppler evaluations of arter-
    ies, 31–33, 39, 43–44
Elastin
    fiber tension, 15, 16–17
    and mechanical properties of
        arteries, 41–42
Enalapril
    affecting brachial artery, 54
    converting enzyme inhibition by,
        51
Endothelin, release of, 49
Endothelium
    age-related changes in, 44
    cholesterol excess affecting, 68
    role in constrictive response, 34
    and vasodilator response to
        increased flow, 17

F

Felodipine affecting blood pressure,
    57

Femoral artery
    compliance and distensibility in,
        40
    diastolic diameter in hypertension,
        33
    mechanical properties in hyper-
        tension, 35
    pulse pressure, 23–24, 30
    in hypertension, 24
Fourier analysis of blood pressure
    curve, 2–4

G

Glucose levels, and arterial stiffness,
    68

H

Heart attack mortality, diastolic and
    systolic pressure curves in, 76
Hemodialysis patients. See Renal
    failure, end-stage
Heterogeneity, vascular, and differ-
    ences in arterial wall structure,
    45
Hydrochlorothiazide
    affecting arterial compliance, 52
    antihypertensive and arterial
        effects of, 57
Hyperemia, reactive, following wrist
    occlusion, 50
Hypertension
    arterial stiffening in, 49
    criteria for diagnosis of, 2, 76
    definitions of, 1–2, 5–6, 76
    long-term drug treatment of, in
        relation to age, 63–67
Hypertrophy of heart. See Ventricu-
    lar hypertrophy

I

Indapamide affecting arterial com-
    pliance, 57–58
Insulin levels, and arterial stiffness,
    68

K

Kidney disease. *See* Renal failure, end-stage

L

Labetalol affecting arterial diameters and compliance, 56
Laplace law, 17

M

Mean blood pressure, 3–4
affecting vascular structure and function, 6–7
calculations of, 4, 5, 11
and cardiovascular risk, 24–25
factors affecting, 13
increased in hypertension, 5–7
Measurement techniques
applanation tonometry, 21–22, 28, 39
echo-Doppler evaluations, 31–32, 39, 43–44
Mechanical properties of arteries, 13, 16–17
age affecting, 35
structural components affecting, 40–41
Media-to-lumen ratio, 61, 62
Metabolic disorders
after antihypertensive therapy, 69
arterial stiffness in, 67–69, 79
Mismatch between heart and vessels, 7, 12, 27
Moens-Korteweg equation, 37, 38
Mulvany-Halpern myograph, 61

N

Nebivol affecting carotid artery distensibility and compliance, 56
Nicardipine affecting arterial diameters, 52, 53
Nicorandil affecting arterial diameter, 53

Nifedipine affecting arterial diameters, 53
Nitrates
affecting arterial diameters, 49, 53–54
affecting arterial dilation and compliance, 17
affecting wave reflections, 30, 59
Nitrendpine
affecting arterial diameters, 53
affecting blood pressure, 57
Nitroglycerin
affecting arterial distensibility, 54
affecting ventricular pressure, 59
Nitroprusside affecting wave reflections, 59
NO, release of, 49
Norepinephrine affecting brachial artery diameter, 56

O

Oscillations around mean pressure, 4, 13

P

Perindopril
affecting arterial structure, 61, 62
affecting brachial artery diameter, 51
affecting cardiac hypertrophy, 62, 63, 64
affecting carotid and femoral compliance and distensibility, 52
converting enzyme inhibition by, 51
Peripheral arteries. *See also* Brachial artery; Femoral artery; Radial artery
diameters compared to central arteries, 33–35, 45
wall structure in, 45
Peterson elastic modulus, 16
in relation to age, 63, 64
Pindolol affecting vascular resistance, 56

Poiseuille law, 5
Pressure-volume relationship, 13–16
Propranolol
    affecting arterial compliance,
        54–55
    affecting wave reflections, 59
Pulsatile arterial hemodynamics,
    58–59
Pulsatility of blood pressure, 4
Pulse pressure, 4, 21–25
    affecting vascular structure and
        function, 7
    age affecting, 25, 63
    arterial changes affecting, 6
    in atherosclerosis, 72
    and cardiovascular risk, 24–25, 77
    characteristics of, 23–24
    determination of, 13
    evaluation throughout arterial sys-
        tem, 23–24
    noninvasive measurements of,
        21–23
    smoking affecting, 68
    in ventricular hypertrophy, 45
Pulse-wave velocity, 37–38
    age affecting, 43
    sodium affecting, 57

R

Radial artery
    antihypertensive therapy affecting,
        62
    compliance and distensibility in,
        39–40
    diameter and wall motion studies,
        32–33
    diastolic diameter in hypertension,
        33
    mechanical properties in hyper-
        tension, 35
    parameters in normotension and
        hypertension, 42
    pulse pressure, 23
        in hypertension, 24
    thickness of, 62
        in hypertension, 43–44

wave reflections related to age, 29
Reflected waves, 25–30
    aortic, age-related increase in,
        29–30
    in atherosclerosis, 72
    backward, 26
    drug-induced changes in, 30,
        58–60
    forward, 25–26
    importance in hypertension, 30
    noninvasive evaluation of, 28–29
    quantification of, 29
    and reflection points near heart,
        27–28
    return during systole, 27, 28
    timing of, 12, 13
        affecting pulse pressure, 6
Renal failure, end-stage
    aortic wave reflections in, 29, 30
    arterial changes in, 69
    pulse pressure measurements in, 23
Resistance, vascular, 11
    in hypertension, 5–6
    increased in middle age, 13
Risk, cardiovascular, and blood pres-
        sure levels, 24–25, 74–76

S

Smoking, and arterial stiffness,
        67–68
Smooth muscle
    age-related changes in, 43
    changes in hypertension, 44
    drug-induced relaxation in, 17, 49,
        53
    and mechanical properties of
        arteries, 41–42
Sodium
    affecting arterial diameter, 56–58
    affecting arterial diameter and
        stiffness, 70
    affecting incidence of strokes, 80
Stiffness of vessels
    affecting diastolic pressure, 12
    aortic, and pulse pressure increase,
        25

in atherosclerosis, 70
Stress affecting arterial wall, 81–82
Stress-strain relationship, 13, 17–19
Strokes, antihypertensive therapy
    affecting, 75, 77, 80
Structural factors
    affecting mechanical properties of
        arteries, 40–41
    and age to begin antihypertensive
        therapy, 81
    antihypertensive drugs affecting,
        61–63
    in central and peripheral arterial
        walls, 45
    mean blood pressure affecting, 6–7
    pulse pressure affecting, 7
    and vascular heterogeneity, 45
Systole, arterial diameter changes in,
    34
Systolic blood pressure
    age affecting, 63, 65
    in atherosclerosis, 70
    and cardiovascular risk, 24–25, 77
    in hypertension, 2
    isolated hypertension, 81
    smoking affecting, 68

T

Tension reduction on arterial walls,
    and capacitance increase, 17
Therapeutic trials
    basic assumptions in, 73–79
    and cardiovascular risk related to
        blood pressure, 74–76
    criteria for entry in, 73, 76
    problems in interpretation of,
        77–79
Thickness of arterial walls
    affecting circumferential stress,
        17–18
    in hypertension, 43–44
Tobacco consumption, and arterial
    stiffness, 67–68

U

Ultrasonography
    echo-Doppler evaluations of arter-
        ies, 31–33, 39, 43–44
    pulse pressure transmission studies,
        24
Unstressed volume, 15–16
Urapidil affecting arterial diameters
    and compliance, 55

V

Vasoactive substances, release of, 49
Vasodilation, and capacitance
    increase, 17
Vasodilator therapy. *See* Antihyper-
    tensive therapy
Ventricular ejection, pulse pressure
    in. *See* Pulse pressure
Ventricular hypertrophy
    increased systolic pressure in, 25
    pulse pressure in, 25, 26, 45
    wave reflections in, 26, 29, 30
Verapamil affecting arterial diame-
    ters, 52
Viscoelasticity of arterial walls, 12
    elastin-collagen ratio affecting, 42

W

Waves
    Fourier analysis of, 4
    propagation of, 12
    reflected, 12, 25–30, 58–60. *See
        also* Reflected waves
Windkessel effect in arteries, 12,
    36–37
Wrist occlusion, reactive hyperemia
    following, 50

Y

Young's modulus of elasticity, 16,
    37, 40, 41–42

u